fit for life

IT HURTS

A PARENT'S GUIDE TO CHILDHOOD
ILLNESSES AND INJURIES

fit for life

IT HURTS

A PARENT'S GUIDE TO CHILDHOOD ILLNESSES AND INJURIES

JANET PODELL &
STEVEN ANZOVIN

Gallery Books
an imprint of W.H. Smith Publishers, Inc.
112 Madison Avenue, New York
New York 10016

A QUARTO BOOK

This edition published in 1990 by Gallery Books,
an imprint of W.H. Smith Publishers, Inc.,
112, Madison Avenue, New York, New York 10016

Gallery Books are available for bulk purchase for
sales promotions and premium use. For details write or
telephone the Manager of Special Sales, W.H. Smith
Publishers Inc., 112 Madison Avenue, New York, New
York 10016. (212) 532-6600.

ISBN 0-8317-3898-7

The information and recommendations contained in this book
are intended to complement, not substitute for, the advice of
your own physician. Before starting any medical treatment,
exercise program or diet, consult your physician. Information is
given without any guarantees on the part of the author and
publisher, and they cannot be held responsible for the contents
of this book.

CONTENTS

COMMON ILLNESSES

ALLERGIES

Allergies are uncomfortable and sometimes dangerous overreactions by the body to irritating substances, called allergens. Children may have allergies to particular foods, inhaled dusts, spores, or pollens, animal hair, substances that come in contact with the skin, or medicines. Allergic reactions may include runny nose and congestion, itching, watery eyes, wheezing and asthma-like symptoms, skin rashes, nausea, vomiting, and, rarely, allergic (anaphylatic) shock.

HAY FEVER
A very common allergy caused by the inhalation of grass or other pollens is hay fever. A child suffering from hay fever will have watery, itching eyes and a swollen, runny nose. Antihistamines taken orally can relieve your child's nasal congestion, but may make your child drowsy. Antihistamine nasal drops and sprays prevent drowsiness, but be very careful not to exceed the recommended dosage.

ANIMAL HAIR, FEATHERS, AND DUST
Common allergens include animal hair, feathers and dust. Exposure to dog or cat hairs or feathers in bedding can cause hay-fever or asthma-like symptoms in some children.

FOOD ALLERGIES
Many children are allergic to certain foods, such as strawberries or shellfish. Symptoms can take the form of hives, vomiting or diarrhea, and wheezing. Headaches, abdominal pains, hyperactivity, and behavioral changes are sometimes blamed on food allergies as well. Unless a definite food allergy has been identified by an allergy specialist, don't exclude too many foods from the diet. Eating a varied diet is the best protection against vitamin deficiencies and other nutritional problems.

ALLERGIC (ANAPHYLACTIC) SHOCK
Some children are dangerously allergic to animal substances (such as bee venom), foods (such as peanut butter), or medicines (such as penicillin). These substances send susceptible children into a form of shock that can be fatal if medical attention is not received immediately. If your child is prone to allergies, have him or her tested by a specialist for dangerous allergies.

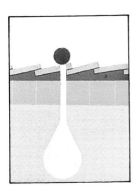 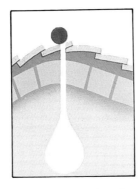 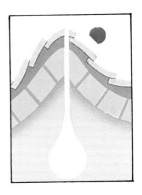

When pollen comes into contact with antibodies in the nasal lining of a hayfever sufferer (1) the excess

fluid that is produced swells the surrounding tissue (2). As part of the body's defense

mechanism, a copious amount of mucus is secreted to disperse the pollen (3).

To treat allergies, skin tests (right) are routinely performed to identify the substances that provoke a reaction.

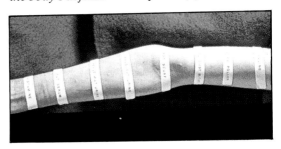

TREATING ALLERGIES

● Hay fever sufferers may benefit from a course of desensitizing injections carried out each winter. See your doctor. Oral and nasal antihistamines are also effective.

● Hair, pollen, and dust allergies can be alleviated by frequent vacuuming of the child's room. Change the bedding often, remove rugs and curtains, and keep pets out.

● Common food allergens include strawberries, shellfish, wheat products, cow's milk and some cheeses, tomatoes, and eggs. Avoid a food if your child has a reaction to it.

● Get medical help immediately if your child loses consciousness after being stung by a bee or wasp or taking penicillin for the first time.

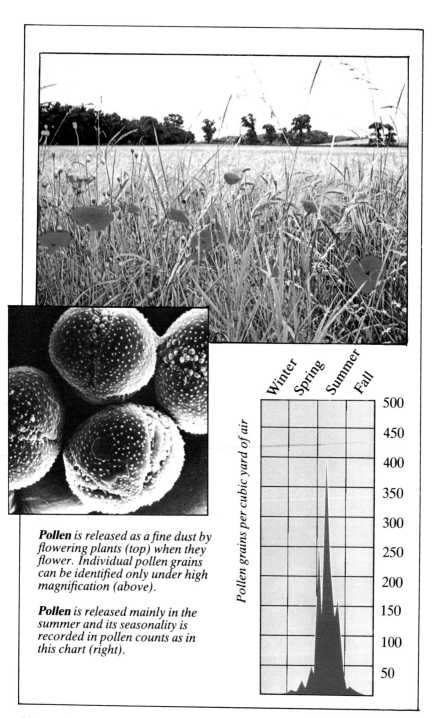

Pollen is released as a fine dust by flowering plants (top) when they flower. Individual pollen grains can be identified only under high magnification (above).

Pollen is released mainly in the summer and its seasonality is recorded in pollen counts as in this chart (right).

ANEMIA

The major function of the red blood cells is to transport oxygen around the body. Red blood cells contain hemoglobin, a red iron-containing substance that picks up oxygen from the lungs and releases it to the body tissues. Hemoglobin, and the cells that contain it, are made in the bone marrow.

Anemia occurs when the blood does not contain enough hemoglobin. Mild anemia does not cause any symptoms, but if it is more severe, the ability of the blood to carry oxygen is impaired. This may cause breathlessness, tiredness, pale skin, and a decreased attention span. One way to tell if your child is anemic is to pinch the child's fingernail and then observe the nail. If it does not immediately turn from white back to pink, but stays white for several seconds, there may be anemia.

Anemia may be due to blood loss, to destruction of the red blood cells by disease, to an inherited defect of the red blood cells, or to an iron deficiency. Too little iron in the diet is the most common cause of childhood anemia in the United States.

IRON-DEFICIENCY ANEMIA

Most children get enough iron in their diets, but some do not. Although most common in toddlers, iron-deficiency anemia can occur at other stages of childhood. The problem can be diagnosed by a doctor with a simple blood test, and treated effectively by giving iron-enriched medicine. The iron in your child's diet can be increased by serving more red meats, fish and green vegetables (especially with citrus fruits, which help iron absorption) and by cooking in cast-iron pots. Do not give your child an iron supplement without asking your doctor; it is also possible to have too much iron in the diet. The recommended daily dietary allowance of iron for 1- to 3-year-olds is 15 milligrams; for 4- to 10-year-olds it is 10 milligrams.

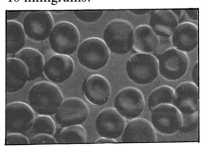

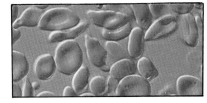

The round disks of red blood cells (left) become distorted in sickle cell anemia (above)

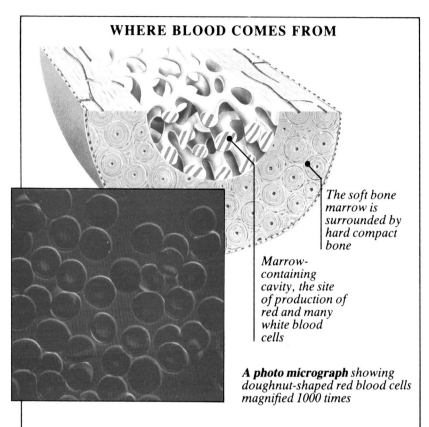

WHERE BLOOD COMES FROM

The soft bone marrow is surrounded by hard compact bone

Marrow-containing cavity, the site of production of red and many white blood cells

***A photo micrograph** showing doughnut-shaped red blood cells magnified 1000 times*

Red blood cells and many white blood cells are manufactured in the bone marrow where they mature before they are carried away to the rest of the body by the circulation of the blood.

Healthy bone marrow that synthesizes blood is a highly active tissue and maintains a constant turnover of blood cells in the body.

SICKLE-CELL ANEMIA

This inherited form of anemia is confined to black children and adults of West African ancestry. Children with sickle-cell disease are more susceptible to infections, are mildly anemic at all times, and may experience sharp pains in the chest, abdomen, and limbs, especially during cold weather. At present there is no cure for sickle-cell anemia, but folic acid, a vitamin, can help the anemia, and aspirin helps the pain.

APPENDICITIS

The appendix is a narrow, blind-ended tube measuring about three inches that arises at the point where the small intestine joins the large intestine. Although it is connected to the digestive system it performs no digestive function in humans. It does, however, sometimes become infected—a condition known as *appendicitis*. The infected appendix swells and, if not removed, may eventually burst, leading to peritonitis, a much more serious infection.

Appendicitis usually starts with abdominal pain centered around the navel. The child loses energy and appetite. The pain usually gets worse over a course of hours. There may be vomiting, a slight fever (100°F or 38°C), and a white, furry coating on the tongue. Gradually the pain moves to the right side of the abdomen. Children complaining of severe and persistent abdominal pain should see a doctor immediately.

The doctor looks for tenderness over the appendix when he or she examines your child. The doctor may then refer your child to a surgeon, because a definite diagnosis is not always easy to make. The doctor may order a blood test and an abdominal X ray to aid in the diagnosis.

Once the diagnosis of appendicitis is certain the appendix should be removed. This operation is called an *appendectomy* and needs to be performed in the hospital. Under general anesthesia, the surgeon cuts off the appendix, the hole in the intestinal wall is repaired, and the incision closed. Children are usually ready to leave the hospital in a few days, but full recovery may take two months or more.

The absence of an appendix appears to cause no problems at all.

The appendix is located at the junction of the small intestine and the large intestine (right).

THE APPENDIX

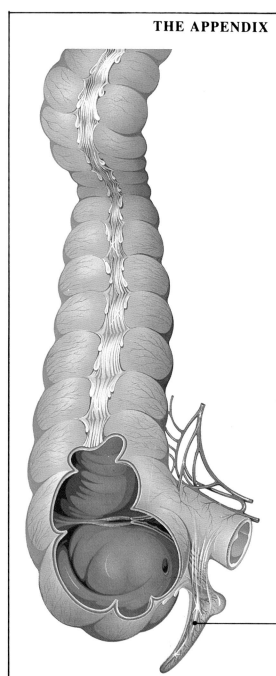

Although the appendix *plays no role in human digestion, the onset of appendicitis makes the sufferer painfully aware of its presence. Approximately the size of an earthworm, the appendix can become blocked and infected, leading to inflammation. If the appendix is not removed in time, it may burst and cause peritonitis—an extremely serious infection. For this reason any child experiencing abdominal pain should be taken to a doctor at once. Happily, the development of peritonitis is very rare and few complications arise from an appendectomy —the relatively simple operation to remove the appendix.*

The appendix

THE DEVELOPMENT OF APPENDICITIS

Appendix opens off colon.

Wall of appendix swells.

Swelling of appendix wall increases.

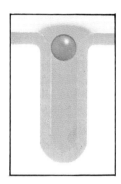
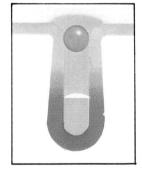
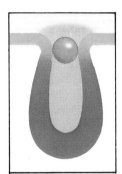

The main telltale signs of appendicitis are:

● pain and tenderness in the center of the abdomen caused by inflammation due to blockage or infection of the appendix

● the gradual localization of pain to the right of the abdomen just above the groin as the inflammation of the appendix increases

● loss of appetite and general nausea

● vomiting, occasionally but rarely persistent

● a fever giving a slightly raised temperature of about 100°F (38.5°C)

Take your child to see a doctor immediately if you are worried about the possibility of appendicitis.

BRONCHITIS AND PNEUMONIA

BRONCHITIS

In toddlers, wheezing may accompany colds and other infections. This is most common in small children who are overweight. The infection starts as a head cold and moves to the chest, causing coughing and wheezing. The child may have some difficulty eating.

These attacks are commonly diagnosed as acute or wheezy bronchitis. Treatment with an antibiotic is the usual course. Improvement occurs in a few days, but such attacks may be the first sign that the child is developing asthma. Bronchitis can also recur through childhood and into adulthood.

PNEUMONIA

An infection of the lung, pneumonia is usually caused by bacteria. This infection may stem from another problem, such as asthma, or from inhaling food or dirty water, or it may follow another infection, such as measles or flu.

The symptoms of pneumonia include coughing and fever. The cough may be dry and hacking, or it may produce a thick green or yellow fluid from the lungs, called sputum. (Children often swallow sputum rather than spitting it out.) Your child may be breathless if the infection is widespread. Other symptoms depend on the particular cause of the infection.

A persistent cough with fever and fluid in the lungs should always be assessed by a doctor. The doctor may find an infection of the

In this X ray of the lungs of a child suffering from pneumonia, the infected area within the right lung can be seen clearly. Breathlessness is a common symptom of pneumonia because the infection interferes with the lung's absorption of oxygen.

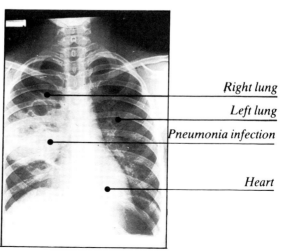

Right lung

Left lung

Pneumonia infection

Heart

CHEST PHYSIOTHERAPY

Chest physiotherapy may be necessary in some cases of pneumonia to drain accumulated mucus from the lungs. The physiotherapist uses a special tapping technique called percussion on the child's chest and back.

lungs when listening to your child's chest. If pneumonia is suspected, the doctor will require a chest X ray to confirm the diagnosis. You can keep a sample of sputum for the doctor to have analyzed at the lab.

Your child will probably be treated with antibiotics. These will clear up the infection in a few days. A hospital stay will probably not be required, except for very young children.

CHICKEN POX

Chicken pox is a highly contagious viral illness characterized by itchy pink pimples. One attack gives a child lifelong immunity to the disease, but the virus may remain in the body in a dormant state and may later cause an outbreak of shingles. Children can catch chicken pox from adults who have shingles as well as from children who have chicken pox.

The incubation period for chicken pox is usually between 13 and 17 days. On the first day of illness, the child has a slight fever and discomfort. Within 24 hours, the rash starts to develop. It starts as small raised red spots which quickly become small blisters and are intensely itchy. After a day or so the fluid in the spots becomes cloudy, a scab forms, and the sore gradually heals.

For the next two or three days new spots continue to appear, so that the rash becomes more severe and extensive. At the height of

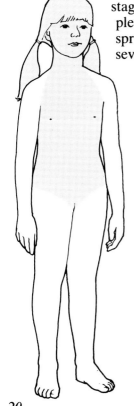

the illness the rash consists of spots at various stages, including red spots, small blisters, pimples, and scabs. The rash starts on the trunk and spreads to the face, the scalp, and the limbs. In severe cases the spots develop inside the mouth, and in girls the groin area may be affected.

While the rash is erupting, the child is ill with a fever, has a poor appetite, and is distressed by the itching. You can apply calamine lotion to soothe the itch.

After about four days have passed, no new spots appear. The child remains infectious until all the spots have scabbed over or disappeared, which takes six or seven days from the start of the rash. In general, chicken pox does not leave permanent scars, unless any of the pimples become infected, usually as a result of scratching.

The itchy spots of chickenpox rash first appear on the face, scalp and body. Within a few days the rash extends to the armpits and groin.

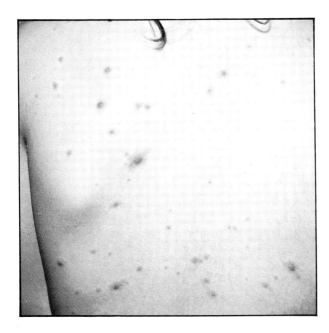

Three or four days after the first symptoms of chickenpox appear, the illness is at its height and all the stages of spot development are present at once (left).

The first spots to appear (right) are small and dark red. These fill with fluid after a few hours to form blisters that eventually dry into scabs. Pink scars are left when the scabs fall off, but these soon fade.

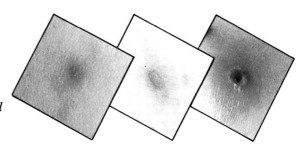

CHICKEN POX

● Chicken pox is a highly contagious disease.

● The first signs of illness are fever and general discomfort, followed by the onset of a rash on the trunk and face.

● The incubation period is two to three weeks.

● Let your doctor know if you think your child is developing chicken pox.

● When the scabs have formed, the child is no longer infectious.

COLDS AND FLU

COLDS

As most people know, there is no cure for the common cold. Colds are caused by viruses; symptoms include a runny nose, watery eyes, sinus congestion, general achiness, and sometimes a slight fever. Colds rarely last for more than four or five days.

Popular home remedies, such as chicken soup, are no more or less effective than anything science has yet devised. Acetaminophen helps control your child's fever and eases the achiness. Hot soup and tea temporarily clear congestion and replace fluids lost through a runny nose. Decongestants clear the nose and sinuses; hot, moist air from a steam vaporizer does the same thing.

FLU (INFLUENZA)

Flus are highly contagious viral infections. They often start with cold-like symptoms, then progress to fever, exhaustion, achiness, and shivering. Flus rarely last more than four to five days.

Each year many new strains of flu arise and sweep through the country, each with slightly different symptoms. Some flu vaccines have been created, but since these treat only a specific flu, they are useless against others that may be going around at the same time. They also have to be given annually. Immunizations against flu are a good idea only for children with heart, lung, or other serious medical problems, to whom an extra illness might be life-threatening. Ask your doctor about it. Healthy children do not need a vaccine.

Bed rest, fluids, and acetaminophen are the best and only treatments for the flu. Watch for possible ear infection or bronchitis afterward.

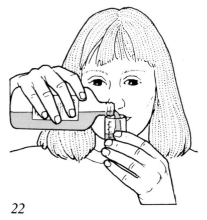

When giving cough medicine to a child it is important to measure out the prescribed dosage precisely. Although it is unlikely that any long-term damage will result from administering more than the recommended amount of a drug, many preparations contain soporifics that may make the child drowsy.

Children's aspirin *will help to alleviate the fever and aches and pains associated with a heavy cold or influenza. To make the tablets more easy to swallow and pleasant to taste they can be crushed between two spoons and mixed with jam.*

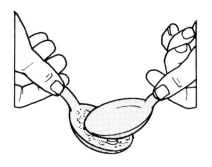

NURSING A SICK CHILD

At some stage almost all parents will need to nurse their child through a cough or cold. *The problem they are most likely to encounter is keeping a restless child who is confined to bed amused. A cuddly toy and a story read aloud are favorite solutions.*

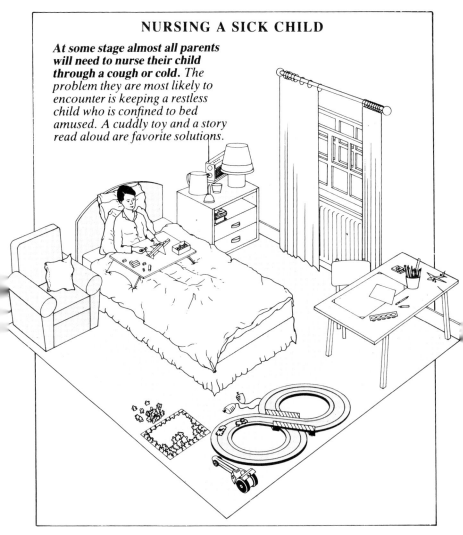

DIARRHEA

The sudden onset of diarrhea in childhood is usually due to infection, either bacterial or viral, or may be caused by eating bad food. It may be accompanied by vomiting. Infectious diarrhea has a short incubation period of one or two days, and because it is highly contagious, several members of the family may be sick at the same time. Diarrhea may be mild—only one or two loose stools—or severe, with so many watery bowel movements that the child quickly becomes dehydrated through loss of fluid. In a dehydrated child, the mouth feels dry, the eyes may appear sunken, and the circulation becomes weak. If this occurs, consult a doctor at once. Dehydration can be fatal in children under two years old.

A toddler with diarrhea should be given plenty of liquid to drink. Many doctors recommend frequent small drinks of cooled, boiled water containing one level teaspoon of sugar and one-half teaspoon of salt dissolved in each pint. If your child is vomiting, or is already dehydrated, the child should be taken to a hospital emergency room immediately and put on an intravenous drip, which brings fluid directly to the bloodstream. Children over two with dehydration, though not in as much danger, should still be given plenty of fluids. Medicines made with kaolin help soothe the intestines and ease the diarrhea, which seldom persists for more than a few hours after fluids are restored.

Since other people may catch the disease from the sick child's stool and vomit, careful hygiene is necessary. The child should be isolated, hands should be washed carefully after toileting, and soiled clothes should be promptly washed.

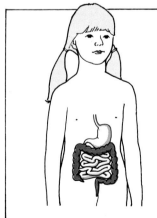

THE DIGESTIVE SYSTEM

Diarrhea is a disorder of the digestive system characterized by frequent watery bowel movements. Viral or bacterial infections of the large and small intestines result in the release of toxins which stimulate more frequent muscle contractions and the secretion of fluid. Inflammation of the mucosa also lessens the absorptive powers of the intestines.

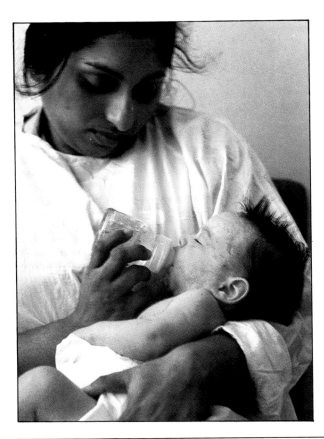

Babies under two years of age are particularly vulnerable to dehydration caused by diarrhea. They may require treatment in hospital, where for the first 24 hours they will be given a clear feed of cooled, boiled water in which a teaspoon of sugar and half a teaspoon of salt have been dissolved.

DIARRHEA

● Infectious diarrhea is highly infectious, with a short incubation period of one or two days. It seldom lasts more than a few days once appropriate treatment has been given.

● Diarrhea is dangerous because it can lead to severe dehydration, especially in children under two.

● Contact a doctor immediately if your child shows the following symptoms:

☛ Very frequent, watery bowel movements.
☛ Pus or blood in the bowel movements.
☛ Fever of 101°F (38°C) or more.
☛ Sunken eyes.
☛ Weak pulse.
☛ Recurrent vomiting.

EAR INFECTIONS

Ear infections may be caused by several different conditions and may affect the ear canal, the eardrum, the middle ear, and the Eustachian tube.

THE MIDDLE EAR

The middle ear in particular easily becomes infected when a child has a cold or other upper respiratory tract infection. In some children the ears are affected every time they have a cold or an allergy attack. Children may also contract ear infections when water enters their ears while swimming. When the middle ear becomes infected the lining membrane becomes thickened and produces a thick secretion. *Otitis media* is the name doctors give to infection of the middle ear.

A child with otitis media complains of discomfort in his or her ear, ranging from a dull ache to acute pain, and loses some hearing in the ear as well. In very young children, look for rubbing or pulling of the ear that may suggest ear infection. Your child will be miserable and irritable if the infection is severe, and there may be a fever and swelling of the neck glands. See your doctor, who will prescribe an antibiotic. The infection usually subsides quickly once treatment has begun. Otitis media can be remarkably tenacious, however, with infections recurring periodically throughout childhood and into adulthood.

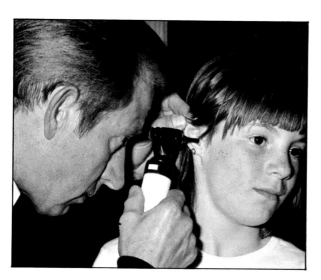

In cases of suspected ear infection, a doctor will use an otoscope to make a thorough investigation. The instrument is placed just inside the child's ear and the examination is completely painless.

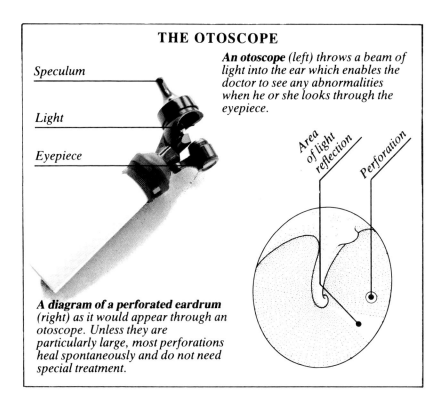

THE OTOSCOPE

Speculum

Light

Eyepiece

An otoscope (left) throws a beam of light into the ear which enables the doctor to see any abnormalities when he or she looks through the eyepiece.

Area of light reflection

Perforation

A diagram of a perforated eardrum (right) as it would appear through an otoscope. Unless they are particularly large, most perforations heal spontaneously and do not need special treatment.

THE OUTER EAR

The outer ear is lined with special skin that produces ear wax. This skin can easily become infected, or affected by other skin diseases. If this happens your child's ear feels blocked or sore, the skin of the ear passage looks red and swollen, and there may be some pus or watery fluid. This is known as *otitis externa,* and it can be treated with antibiotic or anti-inflammatory eardrops.

WAX BLOCKAGE

Children's ears can be gently cleaned periodically to remove excess wax. Wipe away visible wax only; never insert anything into the ear canal, not even cotton swabs, as you could cause damage to your child's ear.

It is not common for children's ears to become blocked by an accumulation of hard wax, but it does sometimes happen. Symptoms can include earache, a ringing in the ears, or even partial deafness. You can remove a blockage of wax under your doctor's direction with an ear syringe containing warm water. Your doctor can remove a stubborn blockage.

EYE INFECTIONS

Contact your doctor if you discover any of the following infections in your child:

CONJUNCTIVITIS (RED EYE)

Conjunctivitis is the commonest eye disease. Inflammation and redness of the eye, with watering and sometimes sticky pus, indicates the infection. Although usually due to a bacterial infection of the eye, conjunctivitis may follow measles or other general infections. Irritation of the eye by chemicals or a foreign particle may also lead to conjunctivitis. Untreated, it can lead to more serious infection of the eye and possibly loss of sight.

Bacterial conjunctivitis is treated with antibiotic eyedrops or eye ointment. Make sure your child keeps his or her hands away from the eyes and washes the hands thoroughly to keep from spreading the infection to the other eye.

STYES

A sty is a localized infection of an eyelash follicle. It looks like a small boil on the eyelid and is uncomfortable rather than painful.

The sty can be treated at home with ointment prescribed by your doctor. Applying moist heat to the inflamed area also helps. Hold a cloth soaked in hot salty water to the sty for a few minutes. This increases the blood supply to the infection and helps it clear more rapidly.

CONJUNCTIVITIS

The red, streaming eyes that are symptomatic of conjunctivitis are a common affliction of childhood. As every parent knows, children are not overly fussy when it comes to washing their hands after playing outside and can all too easily transfer bacteria from their hands to their eyes when they rub them.

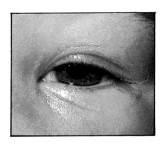

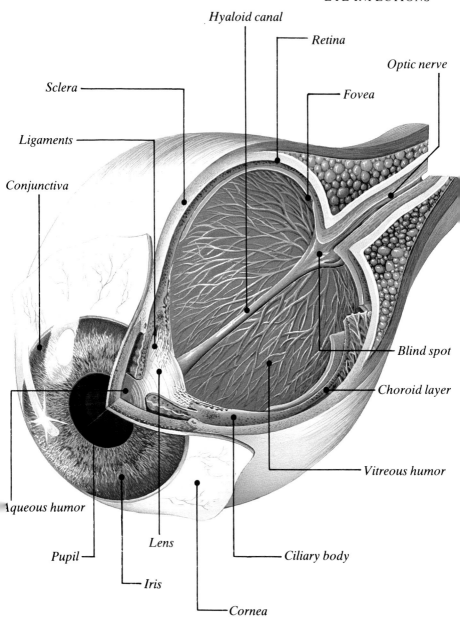

Hyaloid canal

Retina

Optic nerve

Sclera

Fovea

Ligaments

Conjunctiva

Blind spot

Choroid layer

Aqueous humor

Vitreous humor

Pupil

Lens

Iris

Ciliary body

Cornea

Doctors examine the eye *by looking at its movements and the conjunctiva, the cornea, the iris, the lens and the retina. The iris controls the amount of light that enters the* *eye and the lens serves to focus it on the retina where the image is formed and transmitted to the brain via the optic nerve.*

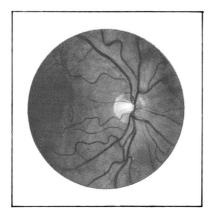

The beginning of the optic nerve, *the retina and the blood vessels that supply it (left) are visible to a doctor using an ophthalmoscope. Sometimes eyedrops that dilate the pupil may be necessary.*

The system of lenses in an ophthalmoscope *(right) help a general practitioner to identify a number of eye disorders and infections. A light shone onto the pupil will reveal whether it constricts properly and whether there is any opacity of the cornea or lens.*

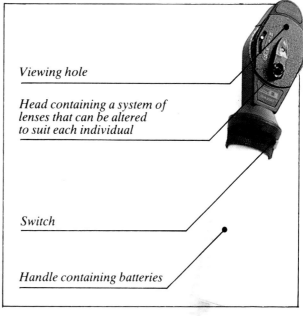

Viewing hole

Head containing a system of lenses that can be altered to suit each individual

Switch

Handle containing batteries

BLEPHARITIS

Blepharitis is an infection of the rim of the eyelids. You can distinguish it from conjunctivitis by the sticky pus accumulating on the eye rim, rather than any redness of the eye itself. Temporarily, your child may lose his or her eyelashes.

Blepharitis is often associated with allergies and dandruff, but it can also be bacterial in origin. Antibiotic ointments work well for the bacterial kinds; ask your doctor about treatment of the other forms of the disease.

FEVER

The temperature of a healthy child is normally between 97 and 99°F (36 and 37°C) during the day. A body temperature above this range usually indicates the presence of an infection. Nearly all common childhood illnesses involve a fever at some point.

When a child's temperature is very high (104°F or 40°C or over), or is persistent, you should consult your doctor to find out the cause and get the appropriate treatment. Whatever the cause, being feverish will make your child feel sick.

FEVER CONVULSIONS
In children five and under, a fever may provoke a convulsion. If your child is convulsing, stay calm. Do not restrain the child. Most fits last less than five minutes and do no real harm. Call your doctor.

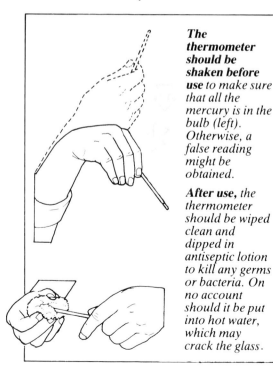

The thermometer should be shaken before use to make sure that all the mercury is in the bulb (left). Otherwise, a false reading might be obtained.

After use, the thermometer should be wiped clean and dipped in antiseptic lotion to kill any germs or bacteria. On no account should it be put into hot water, which may crack the glass.

°F	°C
109.4	43
107.6	42
105.8	41
104	40
102.2	39
100.4	38
98.6	37
96.8	36
95°F	35°C

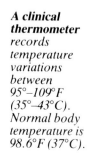

A clinical thermometer records temperature variations between 95°–109°F (35°–43°C). Normal body temperature is 98.6°F (37°C).

TREATING A FEVER

● Lower your child's temperature to make him feel better. If the child feels hot, take off most of his or her clothes and give plenty of fluid to encourage sweating.

● Give acetaminophen (not aspirin for a childhood fever) according to the package directions or your doctor's instructions.

● If the temperature remains high in spite of these measures you can cool your child by sponging the face and body with lukewarm water. This should be done several times, but not for longer than half an hour, or more frequently than every two hours. In the summer, air-conditioning the child's room helps.

● If chills develop, stop the cooling treatment.

TAKING THE TEMPERATURE

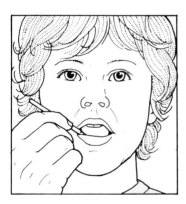 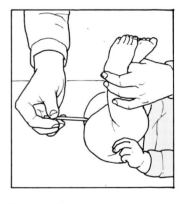

In adults and children the temperature is usually taken by slipping the thermometer under the tongue (above). This method gives the most accurate measurement, but care should be taken to avoid hot or cold drinks immediately before as these may affect the temperature reading.

When taking the rectal temperature, which is advisable in the case of babies (above), a different type of thermometer is used. Naturally, the utmost care should be taken not to push the thermometer in too far.

Sponging your child's forehead has a cooling and soothing effect (right).

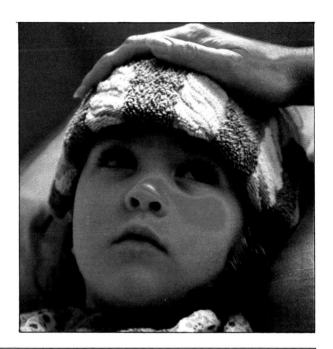

JUNIOR DOSAGE OF ACETAMINOPHEN

AGE	ACETAMINOPHEN IN LIQUID FORM (120mg in 5ml)
1–2 years	5ml of solution (120mg)
2–3 years	5–10ml of solution (120–240mg)
3–5 years	10ml of solution (240mg)

● A doctor might recommend the above doses of acetaminophen to lower a child's temperature, although if the temperature is only just above normal (below 99.5°F/38°C) medication is usually not necessary. If in any doubt about a raised temperature, however, always consult your doctor.

● He or she would probably suggest that the recommended doses are repeated every 6 hours for up to 24 hours. If medication is needed for a longer period, the dosage may need to be reduced. Remember that acetaminophen is potentially dangerous, so be sure to return the bottle to a safe place after each dose.

HEADACHES

Most childhood headaches are not serious and get better quickly. They are often caused by tiredness, and it can be enough just to give your child a snack and a rest. Gently massage your child's face and neck and let the child lie in a quiet, darkened room. Children's acetaminophen will usually take care of any lingering headache.

Some children get more severe headaches, which may be frequent and even disrupt their usual activities. These may be due to migraine or to stress, but there may be other underlying causes for headaches. A headache accompanied by fever is probably due to an infection and a doctor should be consulted.

EYESTRAIN, NASAL AND SINUS CONGESTION, AND ALLERGIES

All may cause headaches. A face and neck rub can be helpful for eyestrain; see an eye doctor to determine if your child needs eyeglasses or a change in the current eyeglass prescription. Decongestants or antihistamines alleviate sinus or allergy headaches. Children who have suffered a head injury may have intermittent headaches for some months afterward, even though there is no lasting damage from the original injury.

If your child is experiencing frequent bad headaches, you may be worried about the possibility of a brain tumor. You may be reassured to know that tumors are rare in childhood and that headaches are seldom the main symptom. More likely, recurrent bad headaches are due to migraine.

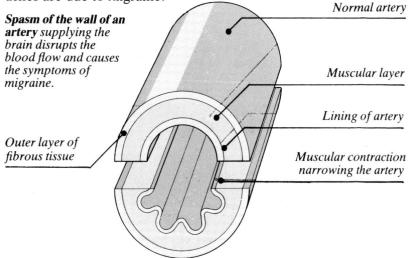

Spasm of the wall of an artery supplying the brain disrupts the blood flow and causes the symptoms of migraine.

Normal artery

Muscular layer

Lining of artery

Muscular contraction narrowing the artery

Outer layer of fibrous tissue

MIGRAINE HEADACHES

In some people, the blood vessels of the brain and scalp can go into spasm, causing migraine headaches. The tendency to migraine headaches runs in families and can be triggered by intense concentration or stress, eating certain foods, or by other still unknown factors. Migraines are excruciating, but splashing ice water on the face and rest in a darkened room make them a little more bearable. Medicines can alleviate some migraine conditions; see your doctor. Older children are more prone to migraine headaches than younger ones.

MIGRAINE

Foods such as coffee, cheese, lemons and chocolate have all been implicated as possible causes of migraine. Other factors, including noise, bright lights, and – most notably – nervous tension are also thought to predispose a susceptible individual to an attack. Once it is obvious that a child is about to have a migraine headache, splashing the face with cold water may help, but by far the best treatment is rest in a darkened room.

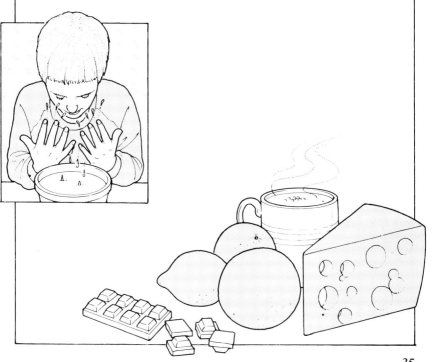

IMMUNIZATIONS

This is the immunization schedule currently used by most pediatricians in the United States.

Age	Vaccine	Method
2 months	DPT (diphtheria, pertussis [whooping cough], and tetanus)	Injection
	Polio	Drops by mouth
4 months	DPT	Injection
	Polio	Drops by mouth
6 months	DPT	Injection
	Polio	Drops by mouth
15 months	MMR (measles, mumps, and rubella [German measles])	Injection
18 months	DPT	Injection
	Polio	Drops by mouth
2 years (18 months if child is in day care)	HiB (hemophilus influenza type B; viral meningitis)	Injection
5 years (before entering school)	DPT Polio	Injection Drops by mouth
10–12 years Girls only	Rubella (German measles)	Injection
14–16 years	DT (diphtheria and tetanus)	Injection
every 10 years in adulthood	DT	Injection

The two most common methods of giving vaccines are by injection (right) or by mouth. Polio vaccine (below) is usually given at the same time as the 'triple' vaccine that provides immunity against whooping cough, diphtheria and tetanus.

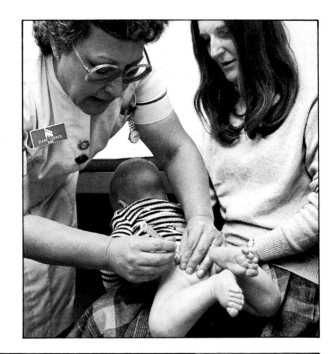

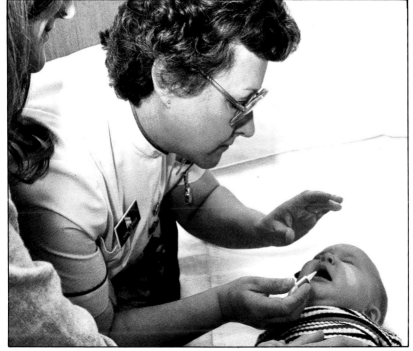

MEASLES

Measles is a highly contagious viral illness. It is characterized by high fever and a rash and may be severe. One attack gives permanent immunity. The incubation period is 10 to 12 days from the time of contact to the onset of symptoms. The child can infect others from the time the first symptoms appear until about five days after the rash has started to come out.

At first, the child has a runny nose (often with bloodstained mucus), a fever, and a dry cough. The eyes may become red with conjunctivitis. A day or two later, tiny white spots appear on the inside of the cheeks and on the back gums.

After two more days, the rash appears. The bigger the rash, the sicker the child will be. The rash consists of dark pink spots which merge to form blotches. It starts behind the ears and across the forehead, then spreads to the front and back of the trunk and the limbs. It lasts for about two days. The child also runs a high fever, up to 105°F (41°C), and has a worsening cough. When the rash starts to fade, the temperature rapidly returns to normal.

Keep the sick child comfortable with bed rest and plenty of liquids to drink. The child may not feel very hungry. Your doctor can suggest treatment for the fever and the cough. If the eyes are affected, the doctor may suggest washing them with warm water. The rash is not itchy and needs no treatment.

Always contact the doctor immediately if you suspect that your child has measles. In some children, the throat, lungs, or ears may become infected. In rare cases, a brain inflammation called encephalitis may develop. Measles can be prevented by a vaccine that is usually given when the child is 15 months old.

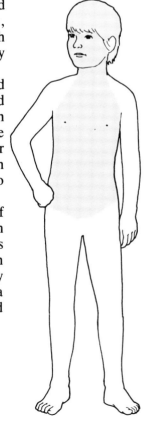

Measles rash *first appears behind the ears and across the forehead, spreading to the front and back of the trunk and finally the limbs.*

SYMPTOMS

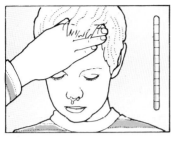

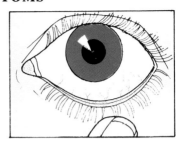

Before the rash appears, a child with measles has the symptoms of a feverish cold.

The child's eyes may become red or bloodshot with conjunctivitis during the first few days.

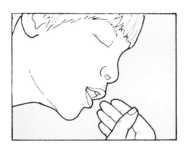

A dry cough and runny nose may also mislead parents into thinking that their child has a cold.

MEASLES

● Measles is caused by a virus that is highly contagious. It is transmitted through droplets from the nose and mouth of an infected person.

● The period between contact with an infected person and the appearance of symptoms is about ten days.

● The first symptoms are fever with a dry cough, red eyes and runny nose. On the second or third day white spots appear in the mouth. On the fourth day a rash breaks out and the fever is high. The rash spreads for several days, then all symptoms subside.

● Keep the child comfortable with plenty to drink. Contact your doctor. Brain inflammation is a rare complication.

● Live measles vaccine given in infancy is effective for many years.

MUMPS

Mumps is a viral disease in which there is tender swelling of the glands just in front of and below the ears. Mumps is less contagious than measles or chicken pox. An attack of mumps gives permanent immunity.

The incubation period for mumps is 14 to 24 days. The illness usually starts with pain and swelling of the salivary glands on the sides of the face. Within a few hours there is a pronounced swelling below the ear, big enough to push the earlobe upward. The swelling extends forward over the lower jaw. There may also be swelling and pain in the glands under the jaw at the front of the neck. One side of the face often swells up a day or two before the other.

The child has a fever, even before the swelling occurs, and suffers pain and general discomfort from the swollen glands. The symptoms gradually subside over four to eight days. Acetaminophen can help reduce the pain. When the swelling has gone down, the child is no longer infectious to others.

Sometimes other parts of the body are affected. The most usual complication involves the brain and its surrounding membranes. This may occur before or after the neck swelling. The child rapidly develops a severe headache and a stiff neck. The temperature rises and the child may vomit. You should consult your doctor immediately if these symptoms occur, whether or not the child has facial swelling.

Children can be immunized against mumps, usually at the age of 15 months.

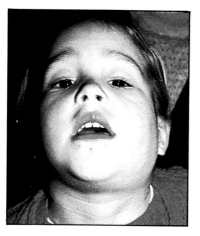

An attack of mumps causes the glands just in front of and below the ears to swell. Often one side of the face swells up a day or two before the other, giving a characteristic lopsided appearance.

If swelling of the parotid gland (A) (right) is pronounced enough it pushes the earlobe upward. The submandibular gland (B), which also swells, is located below the back teeth, under the jaw.

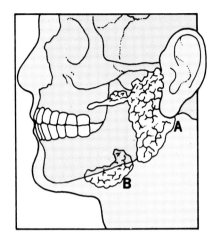

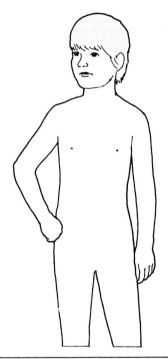

The first unmistakable sign of mumps (left) is usually a swollen parotid gland on one or both sides of the face. The child will run a temperature and be in some degree of discomfort from the swollen glands.
One complication of mumps which occasionally affects adolescent boys is orchitis, pain and swelling in the testicles, which may be accompanied by abdominal pain and nausea.

MUMPS

● Mumps is not highly contagious. Some children will never catch the disease.

● The incubation period is two to three weeks.

● A painful swelling of the neck glands on one or both sides of the face is usually the first sign of mumps.

● This is normally a mild illness, but there are possible complications, such as brain inflammation in children and inflammation of the testicles in adolescent boys and men.

● The child is no longer infectious once the swelling has gone down completely. An attack of mumps gives the child lifelong immunity to the disease.

NAUSEA, VOMITING, AND ABDOMINAL PAIN

NAUSEA
Nausea—queasiness of the stomach—can be caused by eating too much or eating something spoiled. Flus and stomach viruses (gastroenteritis) may make your child feel nauseous, and so can stress, anxiety, dizziness, overexertion, motion sickness, and even sunburn.

VOMITING
Vomiting—emptying of the stomach—often follows nausea, and this is usually a good thing. The body's natural impulse is to reject spoiled food or other noxious substances. Your child will feel much better after vomiting, at least temporarily. Keep your child from swallowing the vomit by having him or her bend forward and vomit into a basin. If the child is lying down, turn his or her head to one side. Generally, call your doctor if your child is vomiting, especially if there is a fever or diarrhea too. For a stomach virus or flu, which may cause repeated vomiting over a 24-hour period, avoid solid food and give clear liquids to prevent dehydration. Your doctor may prescribe dimenhydrinate tablets for motion sickness.

ABDOMINAL PAIN
One of the most common complaints of childhood is abdominal pain. Diarrhea, constipation, urinary infections, and appendicitis may all be accompanied by abdominal pain. Get a medical opinion if your child is suffering from recurrent bouts of abdominal pain, or if he or she is exhibiting other symptoms such as fever, chills, blood in the stool, or vomiting.

Recurrent abdominal pain in children often is due to stress or anxiety. The pain, centering around the navel, may become very severe, making the child cry. It may persist for only a few minutes, or for several hours. After a bout of abdominal pain, children may be well for several months before another bout.

Your child is unlikely to be aware of the cause of his or her inner tension. Stress within the family due to sickness, unemployment, or marital problems can provoke attacks, as can problems at school. Your quiet and sympathetic support is the best treatment. If the pain is severe, your child may want to be in bed; a hot-water bottle is soothing. Acetaminophen also helps with some children.

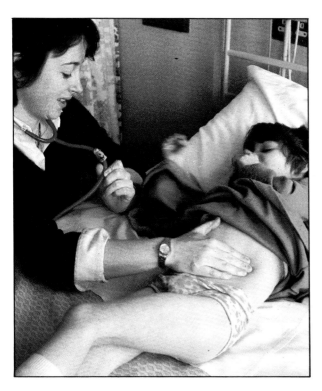

If a child has persistent abdominal pain, *a doctor should be called (left). Before making an examination, he or she will ask about the nature and location of the pain, when the pain started and whether the child has any other symptoms.*

If a child feels nauseous or faint, *he or she should be sat down with the head between the knees and encouraged to breathe deeply (right). Loosen any tight clothing and when the attack is over and the child has recovered give some cold water to drink.*

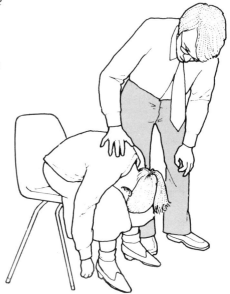

PARASITES

Children of every age and social group may be subject to parasites, tiny animals that live on and in the human body. Parasites can be easily passed from one person to the next, so check all members of your family if you discover parasites on one child. Most parasites can be quickly eliminated with preparation obtained with a doctor's prescription. Contact your doctor if your child has any of the following:

LICE

Head lice are the most common childhood parasite. They are often spread among children at school. Head lice are tiny but visible insects that live on the scalp, sucking blood and causing your child's skin to itch, so that he or she scratches it. The eggs of lice, called nits, are also visible. They look like tiny white or gray grains that are firmly stuck to the hair.

If a child has lice the whole family should be checked and treated if necessary. Treatment is with a special insecticide shampoo that kills both insects and eggs. Wash all clothes and bedding

PINWORMS

These worms infest the rectal area. The major symptom is itching of this area, especially at night. The white, threadlike worms can be seen at night around your child's rectum after the child has been asleep for an hour. Your doctor can prescribe medication that eliminates the worms. Usually everyone in the family must take it at the same time. Wash bedding thoroughly.

TICKS AND CHIGGERS

These are small bugs that burrow into the skin and cause painful itching. They are picked up in wooded areas where children play. If ticks and chiggers are prevalent in your area, dress your child in long sleeves and pants to play outside, and check the child afterwards for bugs clinging to clothes.

Ticks can be removed at home by placing heavy oil or petroleum jelly on the body of the tick. After 15 to 20 minutes it should be possible to withdraw the tick without breaking off the head. Contact your doctor if your child contracts a fever

The bites of chiggers (red mites) cause an itchy rash. Your doctor can prescribe a lotion to kill the chiggers and soothe the itch.

Checking for head lice
is a routine procedure.

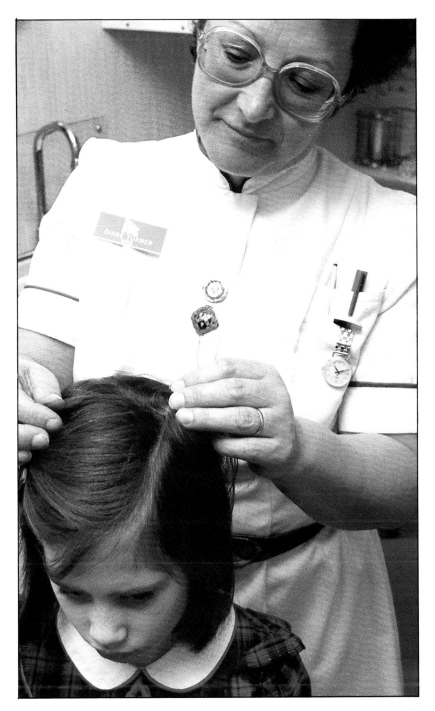

RUBELLA (GERMAN MEASLES)

Rubella (German measles) is caused by a virus. In childhood it is a minor illness, with mild symptoms. However, when a woman in early pregnancy catches German measles, her baby can become infected, and may be born deaf, blind, mentally retarded, or with heart disease. Such babies are usually of low birthweight, and their growth may be stunted. They continue to carry the virus for some years after birth, and can transmit infection to others.

Children who have, or may have, rubella should not be allowed to come into contact with pregnant women. If a pregnant woman suspects that she has the disease, or was exposed to it, she should consult her doctor. A blood test can show whether or not she has been infected.

The incubation period for rubella is two to three weeks. It starts with a runny nose, and the glands in the neck become enlarged. A

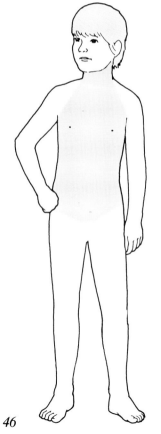

day or two later, the rash appears, starting on the face and spreading down to cover the trunk and limbs over the next 24 hours. The tiny flat pink spots are not itchy and disappear in a day or two. The child remains infectious for up to a week after the start of the illness.

Children can be immunized against rubella, usually at 15 months. In addition, all girls, even those who have had rubella already, should be immunized again during their early teens. Because the disease is mild and therefore difficult to diagnose, doctors can never be absolutely certain that a child has had it, so girls should never assume that they are immune.

A rubella rash usually first appears behind the ears and on the forehead, finally spreading to the trunk.

RUBELLA (GERMAN MEASLES)

● Rubella is a mild infectious disease which does not usually cause children much discomfort. Complications are rare.

● The disease is very dangerous to unborn babies, so it is important for pregnant women to stay away from anyone who may be infected.

● The incubation period is two to three weeks.

● It is a difficult disease to diagnose because symptoms are mild and the rash often disappears before the doctor sees the child. Consult your doctor if you suspect that your child has rubella.

● All girls, even if they have had rubella, should be immunized against it in their early teens.

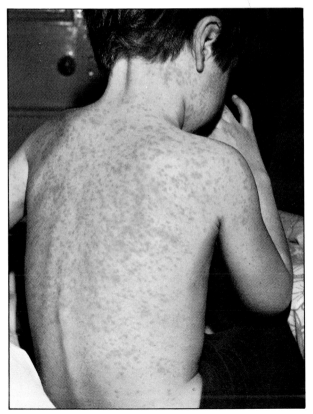

The symptoms of rubella are less severe than measles. The small pink spots typical of the rash (left) do not cause the child any discomfort and usually disappear within a day or two of their appearance.

SKIN DISORDERS

Most children develop skin complaints at one time or another. These may be a rash characteristic of an infection such as measles, or have no obvious cause and disappear by themselves. Common skin disorders include:

COLD SORES (HERPES SIMPLEX)
Cold sores are due to a virus called herpes simplex that infects the skin around the lips and inside the mouth. Some children get cold sores every time they get a cold. At present there is no cure or effective treatment for cold sores. Cold liquids and ice pops ease the discomfort, and so does acetaminophen. The cold sores disappear on their own in a few days.

ECZEMA (ATOPIC DERMITITIS)
Eczema is an itchy, recurrent rash associated with dry skin. Crusty red patches can appear anywhere on the skin. It is often related to allergies, and can be brought on or made worse if your child comes in contact with a substance the child is allergic to, such as wool in clothes. Eczema cannot be cured, but your doctor can prescribe medicines to ease the itch and heal any infections caused by scratching. Avoid drying out your child's skin with harsh soaps; a humidifier in the bedroom can help too.

IMPETIGO
Impetigo consists of red blisters with yellowish crusts. It can be transmitted by contact. Scratching usually makes the infection worse. Antibiotic soaps and oral antibiotics are effective in eliminating impetigo.

PLANTAR WARTS
These warts occur on the bottom of the foot, and can be painful. A foot specialist (podiatrist) can cauterize or remove them.

RINGWORM
Not really a worm, ringworm is a fungus that infects the scalp and sometimes the skin. Look for scaling and patches of broken hair on the scalp, or characteristic red, ring-like patches on your child's skin. Ringworm is easily passed from person to person, and also from and to animals. Your doctor can prescribe an effective treatment for the fungus.

KEEPING BABY CLEAN

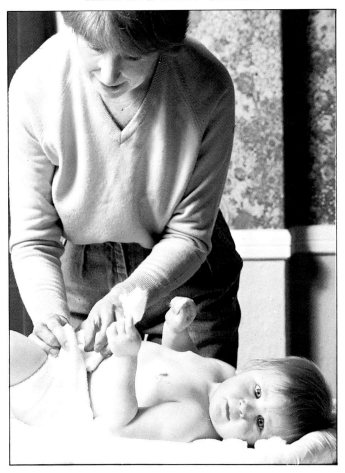

Because a baby has less resistance to infections and skin complaints than an older child or adult, it is important to pay scrupulous attention to keeping your baby clean. Diapers should be changed frequently and the diaper area washed with tissues or cotton wool moistened with water or baby lotion. After drying the baby thoroughly a barrier cream should be applied if there is any redness or sign of irritation. If, even after your best efforts, diaper rash occurs, by far the most effective treatment is to leave your baby's diaper off and let exposure to the air do its healing work.

SORE THROAT

Many illnesses have a sore throat as one of their symptoms. These include colds, flu, tonsillitis, mumps, and ear infections.

Treatment of sore throat begins with trying to determine its cause. Check other sections of this book for clues to diagnosing the illnesses listed above. For any case of very painful sore throat accompanied by fever and vomiting, or if you think your child may have inhaled smoke or a poison, see your doctor.

STREP THROAT

One of the most common causes of sore throat are bacteria, called streptococcus, that infect the throat and ear. Strep throats are quite painful. Your child may complain of throat pain and have trouble swallowing. Look for a sudden fever, weakness, and possibly vomiting. Your child's tongue will have a white, furry coating with tiny red dots, and the throat will look red and inflamed. Contact your doctor, who will probably prescribe an antibiotic to kill the infection. Give the full course of treatment even though your child feels better in a day or two. Cold liquids and ice cream temporarily ease the throat pain. Be alert for a possible ear infection following a strep throat.

SCARLET FEVER

Scarlet fever is also caused by the streptococcus germ. It starts like a strep throat, but a day or two later a bright red rash spreads from your child's neck down to the entire body. Antibiotics are equally effective in treating scarlet fever.

In the past, rheumatic fever and kidney damage sometimes followed a strep infection. These are now very rare, and do not occur in children who receive prompt treatment.

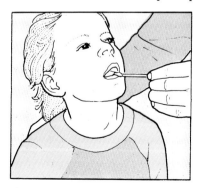

If it is thought that a child suffering from a sore throat has an infection, a swab will be taken for analysis in the laboratory. A sterile cotton bud is rubbed gently over the site where the infection is suspected.

TONSILLITIS

The tonsils are swellings of tissue on each side of the back of the throat. They grow rapidly in early childhood and reach a peak in size around age five before gradually shrinking back in size during later childhood.

TONSILLITIS

Your child's tonsils may become infected by bacteria or viruses, causing a sore throat, a condition called tonsillitis. An upper-respiratory viral infection may affect the tonsils, but such an infection does not require specific treatment and passes in a few days. More serious are bacterial infections, with a sore throat, difficulty in swallowing, and possibly a fever. Your child's throat looks bright red and there may be some pus on the surface of the tonsils. The child's neck glands (lymph nodes) may be swollen. See your doctor if these symptoms are present. Usually, treatment with an antibiotic begins to clear up the infection within 24 hours.

TONSILLECTOMY

Some children are prone to recurring attacks of tonsillitis. Often a prolonged course of antibiotics clears up tonsillitis for good. But if the tonsils become the focus of continuing infections, and sore throats are frequent, your doctor may recommend that your child's tonsils be removed by a surgeon. This operation is called a *tonsillectomy*. With your child under an anesthetic, the surgeon carefully cuts away the infected tonsils. (Sometimes the adenoids, tissue areas at the back of the nasal cavity that are also prone to infections, may be removed at the same time.) Following the operation your child's throat will be sore for a few days—ice cream is the recommended therapy—but recovery is rapid.

The tonsils at the back of the mouth form part of the body's defence system. Infection may cause them to become inflamed and a child who has a sore throat frequently could probably benefit from having a tonsillectomy.

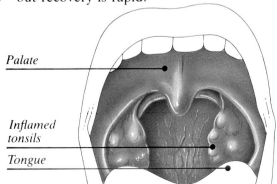

Palate

Inflamed tonsils

Tongue

TOOTHACHE

Most toothaches are caused by decay that has eaten a hole, or cavity, through the tooth into the nerve at the center. A child who has a toothache should be taken to a dentist right away. At night, or if a dentist is not available, first aid treatment may be necessary. You can dip a cotton swab into oil of cloves and insert it gently into the cavity to temporarily relieve the pain. (Oil of cloves is available at drugstores and should be kept with your first aid kit.) Be sure that the oil does not touch anywhere except the cavity. If you have no oil, or if no cavity can be seen, trying giving your child ice to suck. Aspirin or acetaminophen may also give some relief.

The best way to prevent toothache is good oral hygiene and feeding your child nutritious food. Foods containing sugar, honey, corn syrup, and other sweeteners make the child's mouth an ideal place for bacteria to grow. These bacteria eat away the enamel on the outside of the tooth. If the cavity is not filled by a dentist, the bacteria attack the rest of the tooth, which may eventually be lost. Giving your children fruit rather than cookies and candy can help keep their teeth healthy.

Daily care of the teeth is also important. Parents should begin brushing their children's teeth in infancy with a soft brush that has a small head. Most dentists recommend that you use a back-and-forth movement for the chewing surfaces of the teeth and an up-and-down movement for the other surfaces. Regular visits to the dentist can help catch problems before they get worse.

Fluoride has been found to prevent tooth decay when taken in minute quantities. If your drinking water does not have fluoride added to it, your dentist may suggest that you give your child fluoride drops or tablets.

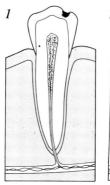
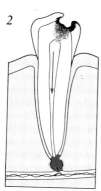

Sugary foods and inadequate dental hygiene contribute to tooth decay. Bacteria left in the mouth form plaque which erodes enamel (1) and attacks the dentine underneath. If the cavity that results extends to the pulp cavity, which contains a nerve, toothache is the inevitable consequence (2).

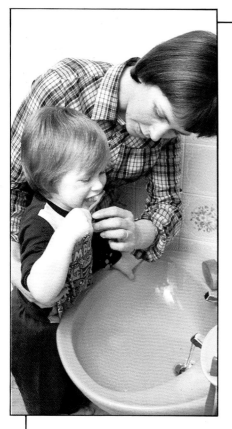

DENTAL CARE

Proper care of the teeth should begin at the earliest possible age. Good habits last a lifetime, and a child should be taught the importance of regularly brushing their teeth to avoid decay. By making dental care fun rather than an unpleasant chore the child is less likely to resist attempts to get him or her to clean the teeth after meals.

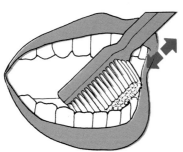

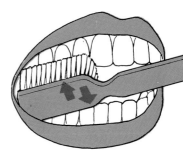

Preferably, use a brush with a small head to clean the teeth. The front top and bottom teeth should be cleaned with a vigorous up and down motion,

making sure that any gaps between teeth are not forgotten. The back teeth, chewing and inside surfaces can then be tackled.

53

URINARY TRACT INFECTION

Infection of the urinary tract is common at all ages. It is caused by bacteria that normally live harmlessly in the intestines. Sometimes these bacteria enter the urethra (the opening through which urine passes out of the body). If they can overcome the body's natural defenses, they travel to the bladder and cause an infection known as cystitis. They may then spread further up the urinary tract to affect the kidneys. Girls are much more prone to urinary tract infections than boys because the urethra is shorter in females.

In children past infancy, the infection may start suddenly or may come on so gradually that the symptoms are barely noticeable. If it starts suddenly, the child may run a high fever, up to 105°F (41°C), accompanied by attacks of violent shivering. Poor appetite, nausea, vomiting, diarrhea, and blood in the urine are all common in severe acute urinary tract infections. If the onset of infection is more gradual, the child may experience pain when urinating or abdominal pain just after urinating, and may have a poor appetite and general listlessness. In most cases the child feels the need to urinate frequently. A child who is ordinarily dry through the night may wet the bed.

The doctor makes a full examination of a child with these symptoms. A clean specimen of urine is sent to the laboratory, where it is checked under a microscope and cultured to see if there are any bacteria present. When the results are known, the doctor selects

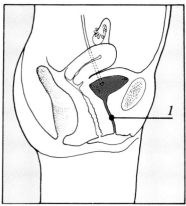 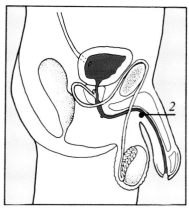

The bacteria that are the normal inhabitants of the bowel may overcome the body's defences and pass up the urethra to the bladder *and cause an infection. Girls (1) are more susceptible to urinary tract infections than boys (2) because their urethra is shorter.*

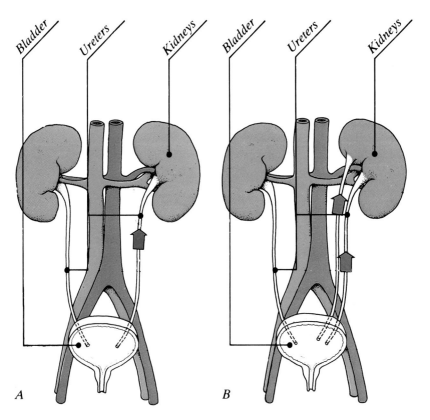

Bladder Ureters Kidneys Bladder Ureters Kidneys

A B

Urine (A) is usually prevented from flowing upward by the valves that connect the ureters to the bladder. If the valves do not function properly, emptying the bladder may cause a backflow of urine and the development of an infection. If the infection is not diagnosed and treated at early enough stage, it may spread and damage the kidneys.

A relatively common congenital abnormality (B) is the presence of an extra, or double, ureter. Because the flow of urine is divided into two and consequently reduced, the individual is more prone to urinary infection. The arrows indicate how the infection spreads, which is fastest inside the double ureter.

the most appropriate antibiotic drug, which is usually taken by mouth for at least ten days. Give your child plenty of liquid to drink. This helps to wash out some of the bacteria every time the bladder is emptied.

After the treatment is finished, the doctor sends follow-up specimens to the laboratory to make sure that the infection is gone. The doctor may also arrange for X rays of the urinary tract and for an ultrasound picture of the kidneys to be taken. (Note that some children are dangerously allergic to the X-ray dye.)

WHOOPING COUGH (PERTUSSIS)

Whooping cough, also known as pertussis, is a highly contagious disease caused by bacteria. The infection produces a sticky mucus that blocks the lungs and windpipe, making it hard for the sick person to breathe. The disease can affect people of all ages but is most serious in babies and young children. It has an incubation period of one to two weeks.

At first the child appears to have a cold, with coughing, a slight fever, and a runny nose. This is the stage at which the child is the most infectious, and it lasts for about a week. Gradually the cough gets worse and starts to come in spasms. During a bout of coughing the child cannot breathe and turns red or blue in the face. It is a frightening feeling, and a parent's touch is very comforting. When the spasm is over, the child may vomit up sticky mucus. Firm banging on the child's back may help in bringing up the mucus. The child's breathing afterwards may be noisy—the so-called 'whoop'. The worst coughing usually occurs at night. The coughing is so violent that the child's eyes turn red from broken blood vessels.

Bursts of coughing, accompanied by choking and vomiting, may persist for two or three months. Even when whooping cough appears to be getting better, symptoms may become much worse again if the child gets a secondary infection such as a cold.

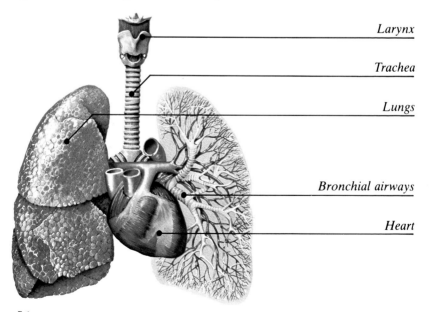

Larynx

Trachea

Lungs

Bronchial airways

Heart

WHOOPING COUGH

● Whooping cough is a highly infectious disease that can be prevented by a series of immunizations. It forms part of the DPT shot, along with diphtheria and tetanus.

● The disease starts with a runny nose and a slight cough. The more serious symptoms develop in about a week. The cough gradually gets worse, occurring in violent spasms, followed by loud breathing and vomiting of mucus.

● Symptoms can persist for three to four months. There is no effective medicine.

● The disease can be very serious, particularly for children under the age of two.

There is no effective treatment for whooping cough. Antibiotics have no influence once the symptoms appear.

Children can be immunized against pertussis. Most pediatricians recommend a series of vaccinations, beginning with three during the first year of life, with booster shots given periodically afterward. The vaccination may cause fever and crankiness. In very rare cases, children have severe reactions to the vaccination and suffer brain damage. Your doctor can explain the safety issues.

HOME NURSING OF WHOOPING COUGH

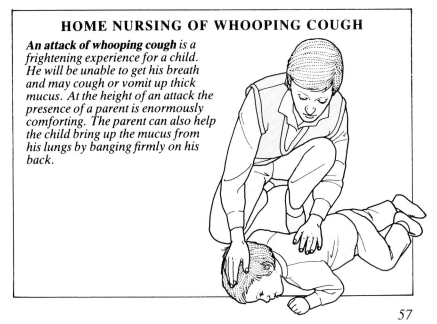

An attack of whooping cough is a frightening experience for a child. He will be unable to get his breath and may cough or vomit up thick mucus. At the height of an attack the presence of a parent is enormously comforting. The parent can also help the child bring up the mucus from his lungs by banging firmly on his back.

COMMON INJURIES

BITES

Bites can be dangerous wounds. They can quickly become infected, especially human bites. Seek immediate medical attention for any bite that breaks the skin. If it is from an animal, try to capture or identify the animal for examination.

SNAKE BITES

The bite of a poisonous snake can be distinguished from the bite of a nonpoisonous snake by the prominent fang marks at the front of the bite. Snake bites are of varying severity, depending on the kind of snake, the amount of venom injected, and the victim's age and health. Poisonous snake bites in children are very serious. Symptoms may include swelling and redness at the bite, nausea, vomiting, dizziness, slurred speech, convulsions, and paralysis. Get medical help immediately. Give first aid as described here.

TREATMENT FOR DOG AND OTHER ANIMAL BITES

● Wash the wound with water and mild soap until it is clean.

● Look carefully for penetrating wounds that may be difficult to clean.

● Apply a clean, unmedicated dressing.

● Take the child to a doctor or the nearest hospital for assessment of the bite and for a tetanus shot if none has been given in the last two years.

● Human bites should be treated as for dog bites. These are very likely to become infected and must be seen by a doctor.

TREATMENT FOR SNAKE BITE

● Immobilize the bitten part to slow down absorption of the venom. Do not let your child walk around. If necessary, carry the child to help.

● Cover the bite with a dry dressing.

● Transport to the hospital immediately, preferably in a lying position. Use CPR techniques if your child stops breathing. *Do not* apply a tourniquet, suck out the poison with your mouth, cut the wound to make it bleed, or apply any chemical to the bite.

● Nonpoisonous snake bites can be treated like other animal bites.

BROKEN BONES

In childhood, broken bones (fractures) are usually caused by falls, while playing sports, or in road accidents. Arm, leg, finger, toe, and collarbone fractures are the most common.

Fractures in children do not always extend right across the bone, but may crack only one side. This is called a greenstick fracture. A fracture that does not break the skin is a closed fracture. If the skin is broken it is called an open or compound fracture, and there is a risk of infection.

Suspect a fracture after a fall or injury if your child has pain, swelling, deformity of a bone or joint, or is unable to use the limb. Take your child to an emergency room, where an X ray will be taken, the bones set, and often a cast fitted on the fracture. Leg injuries may need to be immobilized by traction, and collarbone fractures will need to be treated with a special sling. Broken fingers and toes may be splinted to the adjoining digit, or simply left to heal by themselves.

PREVENTING BROKEN BONES
As for most injuries, the best first aid for broken bones is prevention: Drive carefully and defensively; keep low windows shut or install safety bars on them; fit a safety gate to stairs to stop toddlers falling; teach your child traffic safety rules; don't enroll your children in violent sports, such as football or karate, before they are physically mature enough.

Collar bone fractures do not usually result from direct pressure, but from a fall on the hand or on the shoulder that causes the force of the impact to travel up the bone. Ankle fractures most often result from the leverage exerted when a fall twists the ankle. Fractures may also occur from direct impact, for example an arm broken by a blow from a heavy object.

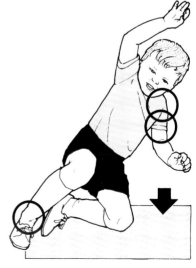

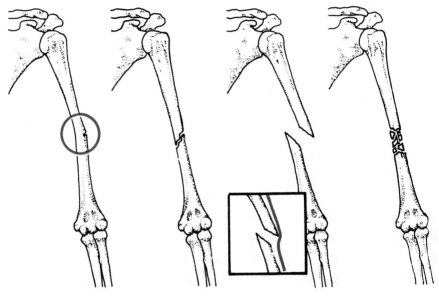

In a greenstick fracture the bone is only partly broken on one side.

The bone does not protrude through the skin in a closed fracture.

The surface of the skin is broken in a compound fracture.

In a comminuted fracture the bone is broken into several pieces.

FIRST AID FOR BROKEN BONES

● Get emergency help immediately for an open fracture or a broken neck or spine—these are possible in any car accident or fall from a height. Do not move the child yourself unless there is immediate danger—if the child is lying on the road, for example.

● Perform the minimum of first aid yourself. You can make a sling for a broken arm, but leave broken legs, ribs, hips, and skulls alone until help comes. You can take a child with a broken arm, jaw, collarbone, wrist, ankle, finger, or toe to the hospital yourself.

● Treat for shock if necessary (see 'Shock' in this book).

● Do not give the child liquids or food in case general anesthesia is required later.

BRUISES AND SCRAPES

Children collect bruises and scrapes as a part of growing up. Like minor cuts, most of these heal with no attention from you (other than a little comforting).

BRUISES
A bruise results when blood vessels have been broken under the skin by a blow or impact. The bruise will swell and change color from red to blue–black to yellowish. Bruises generally disappear after a few days. Fair-skinned children in particular are likely to spend their childhood with bruises up and down their legs acquired in everyday playing.

Quick application of a cold compress helps reduce the swelling. Inspect for possible bone or other damage at the bruise site. If you think there may be an internal injury, contact your doctor.

A recurrent pattern of bruises, especially on the body or face, may indicate that your child is being abused. Ask your child about bullying at school or from an adult; no matter how reluctant the child is to discuss it, usually you can get some clue to the problem. Talk to your doctor.

SCRAPES
Many scrapes can be avoided by dressing your child in long sleeves and pants when the child is playing on asphalt or concrete. Helmets, elbow and knee protectors, and riding gloves protect children who like to 'stunt ride' on their bicycles or play with skateboards.

When presented with a scrape, inspect it for embedded dirt or gravel. Rinse the scrape under cold water to wash these away. Your child can help by dabbing carefully with a clean cloth to dislodge stubborn particles.

Scrapes where particles have been forced under the skin and can't be removed, or where a large area of skin has been abraded away, should be seen by a doctor.

BURNS

Burns are caused by skin contact with flame, hot objects or harsh chemicals. As with other injuries, the best way to deal with burns is to prevent them.

● Keep small children away from stoves and ranges. Don't let pot handles extend within reach of a child.
● Teach your children respect for fire. Don't leave matches within reach.
● Store harsh or dangerous chemicals in a locked cabinet.

The seriousness of a burn depends on the size of the area burned and the depth of the burn. Any burn that covers more than 10 per cent of your child's body or that appears to penetrate into the skin must be seen by a doctor immediately.

BURN TYPES
Burns are classified into three general types:
1st-degree burns are relatively mild. They tend to be small in area, red or discolored, mildly painful, and heal quickly. Sunburn is classified as a first-degree burn.
2nd-degree burns are more serious, and often the most painful. The burned area penetrates deeper into the skin, looks red, mottled, and wet, develops blisters, and swells over a period of days.
3rd-degree burns are always serious. They completely destroy body tissue. They are deep, look white or charred, and result in the destruction of the skin in the burned area.
Chemical burns can look like any of the above. In addition, the skin may absorb the chemical, which can lead to poisoning.

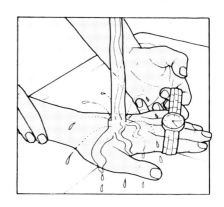

Immediate first aid for a burn involves immersing the affected area in cold water to cool the tissues and prevent further injury. Any constricting jewelry or clothes should be removed to prevent swelling. Blisters should not be broken or the burnt area touched. A sterile dressing secured by a loose bandage should be applied after the injury has been cleaned.

FIRST AID FOR BURNS

1st DEGREE
- Immediately run cold water over the burned area. Apply cold cloths.
- Gently bandage with gauze. Do not use ointment or cream,
- Do not break any blisters that develop.

2nd DEGREE
- Treat as for 1st-degree burns and see your doctor.

3rd DEGREE
- Get medical help immediately.
- Lay your child down. Do not remove burned clothing or touch the burn.
- Gently cover the burn with a loose sterile dressing.
- Treat for shock (see 'Shock' in this book).

CHEMICAL BURNS
- Get medical help immediately.
- Rinse the burned area with cool water for at least five minutcs. Remove contaminated clothing during the rinse.
- Follow the first-aid instructions on the chemical container, if any.

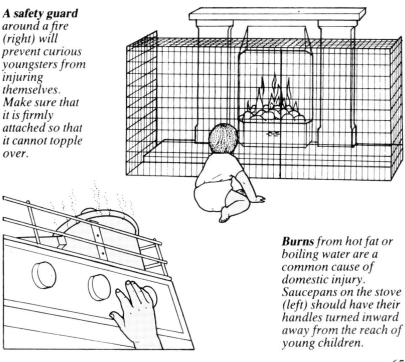

A safety guard around a fire (right) will prevent curious youngsters from injuring themselves. Make sure that it is firmly attached so that it cannot topple over.

Burns from hot fat or boiling water are a common cause of domestic injury. Saucepans on the stove (left) should have their handles turned inward away from the reach of young children.

CHOKING

Choking occurs when the airway is partly or totally blocked and the child cannot breathe. It is one of the leading causes of accidental death in children, especially children under the age of four.

PREVENTING CHOKING
Most choking incidents can be prevented by the following measures:

● Keep small objects that can be swallowed away from infants, toddlers, and small children. Teach older children not .to put foreign objects in their mouths and not to give them to smaller children.

● Buy sturdy toys that cannot be broken into small pieces that could be swallowed.

● Avoid serving whole nuts, hard candy, whole carrots, fruit with pits, whole hot dogs or sausage, or other unchopped meat to small children.

● Teach children to eat slowly, chew thoroughly, and not to talk when food is in their mouths. Set a good example yourself.

TREATING CHOKING
Most choking incidents end quickly with the child coughing up the obstruction unaided. As long as your child can breathe or talk, be alert but do not take the following steps. If the child cannot breathe, you have to take action at once. It is essential that any obstruction in the airway be removed immediately.

A child who is choking needs immediate first aid. After removing any obstruction from the mouth, the child should be lain over a knee and slapped sharply between the shoulder blades.

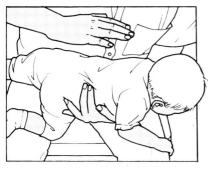

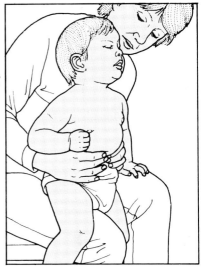

Babies are particularly vulnerable to choking because they lack the reflexes to dislodge the obstruction themselves. A choking baby should be held downward, with the chest and abdomen supported. If sharp taps between the shoulder blades do not work, sit the baby on your lap. Place two fingers from each hand just above the baby's navel and press firmly upwards.

CHOKING FIRST AID

● Watch for signs of violent choking—clutching the throat, crowing or strangled sounds, blueness in the face, neck, and hands (cyanosis).

● Quickly remove any objects or fluids from your child's mouth. Lay the child over your knee with the head down. With one hand support the chest and with the other slap the child briskly between the shoulder blades, up to four times. If this doesn't work—

● Stand behind your child and wrap both arms around the stomach between the navel and the rib cage. Clasp your hands together and make four upward thrusts. (This technique is sometimes called the Heimlich maneuver.) Gauge the amount of force you use to the size of the child. The obstruction may be expelled forcefully from the mouth.

● If your child is unconscious, place the child on a firm surface and roll him or her onto one side. Slap twice between the shoulder blades. Check to see if the obstruction has been dislodged. Give CPR and get emergency medical help immediately.

CPR (CARDIOPULMONARY RESUSCITATION)

Cardiopulmonary resuscitation is a rescue technique that can save the life of a child who stops breathing or whose heart stops beating. You must start this technique immediately. It takes only three minutes for brain damage to occur in a person who has stopped breathing.

The two key factors to check before beginning CPR are: Is the child still breathing? Has the heart stopped?

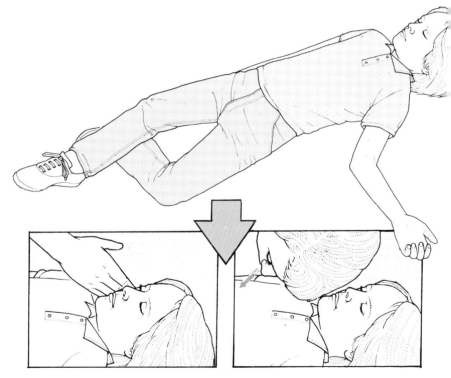

If you get no response from tapping the child's face, check whether they are breathing. **Watch** *to see if the chest and abdomen rise and fall and listen at the mouth. If there is no evidence of breathing follow the steps opposite.*

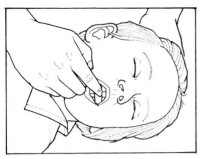

With the child on his back *turn the head to one side and clear the mouth of any obstruction, such as blood, vomit or other objects.*

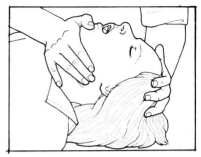

If the child is still not breathing, *tilt the head back, holding the forehead and chin, and open the mouth to begin artificial respiration.*

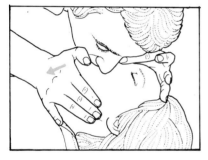

After taking a deep breath, *pinch the child's nostrils closed and place your mouth over the child's. Give five short breaths.*

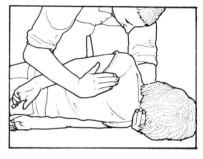

If the chest does not rise, *pull the child toward you so that he is on his side and slap him twice between the shoulder blades.*

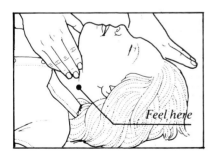

Feel here

If you can feel a pulse *on the child's neck, give two breaths into his mouth. If there is no pulse start heart massage.*

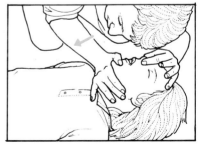

Continue breathing into his mouth *every five seconds until breathing starts or medical aid arrives. Place the child in the recovery position if breathing does restart.*

CUTS AND WOUNDS

For the many minor cuts and wounds your child incurs, the best approach is to do as little as possible. Most small cuts, if kept dry and clean, heal by themselves with no problem. Use a breathable adhesive bandage to keep the cut clean, but do not apply an antiseptic cream or ointment, which only retards the healing process.

JAGGED WOUNDS

Rinse jagged wounds under running water to make sure that no dirt remains. Flaps of skin should be left in place to heal back together or drop off on their own. If a foreign object is buried too deeply under the skin to remove, see your doctor. Any large wound that may need stitches should be seen by a doctor

PUNCTURE WOUNDS

Needle, pin, or thorn punctures quickly heal by themselves. Punctures with a rusty nail, spike, or tool should be seen by a doctor. Keep your child's tetanus immunizations up to date.

MAJOR CUTS AND WOUNDS

The primary objectives with a major wound are to stop the loss of blood and to get medical help immediately. Take the steps listed here.

INTERNAL BLEEDING

Look out for signs of faintness, rapid pulse, cold sweaty skin, thirst, or rapid breathing. These could be signs of internal bleeding. Get medical help immediately.

FIRST AID FOR SERIOUS BLEEDING WOUNDS

1 Apply firm, prolonged pressure over the wound after first removing any obvious foreign bodies.

2 If the wound is large, press the edges together gently and maintain pressure.

3 If possible, lower the child's head and raise the bleeding part.

4 Cover the wound with a sterile dressing. Cover the dressing with a soft pad and tape in place.

5 If you child has lost a lot of blood, treat for shock.

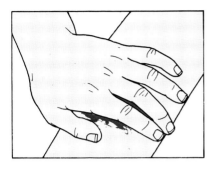

Apply prolonged pressure *over the wound after first removing any obvious foreign bodies.*

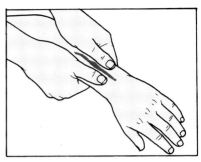

If the wound is large, *press the edges together gently and maintain pressure.*

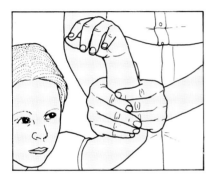

If possible, *lower the child's head and raise the bleeding part.*

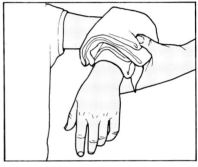

Prepare a sterile dressing *that will easily cover the wound. Cover with a soft pad and bandage firmly.*

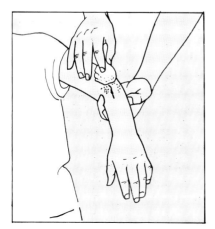

In the case of minor bleeding, *apply an antiseptic lotion to the wound repeatedly until any visible dirt particles have been washed away. A large sterile dressing should then be applied to cover the wound.*

EYE INJURIES

CUTS ON THE EYE
If your child's eye has been cut or penetrated by a sharp object, such as flying glass, take the child to an emergency room immediately. Do not try to remove the object yourself. Tape a paper cup over the eye with cloth tape to keep your child from rubbing the eye and injuring it further.

CHEMICAL BURNS ON THE EYE
If the eye has been burned by a chemical such as acid, hold your child's head under cold water for several seconds or pour water over the eye with a pitcher. Make sure the child blinks and opens the eye while you are doing this. Take the child to an emergency room immediately while continuing to wash the eye if possible.

REMOVING SMALL PARTICLES IN THE EYE
Small particles in the eye must be removed as soon as possible to avoid damage to the surface of the eye. Tears help to float out particles. Keep your child from rubbing the injured eye—suggest that the child rub the *other* eye, which will encourage tears in both.

BLACK EYE
A black eye is actually not an eye injury, but a bruise to the bone and tissue surrounding the eye. Reduce swelling and pain with a cold compress. See your doctor if you think there has been any serious damage to the area around the eye.

REMOVING PARTICLES FROM THE EYE

● Put your child under a good light and lift off the particle with the moistened tip of a clean cloth or tissue.

● If the particle is stuck under the upper lid, gently hold back the lid and, with the child looking down, rub it gently over the lower lid.

● If this doesn't work, a matchstick may be placed in the fold of the upper lid and the eyelid pulled up over it. Remove the particle with the tip of a moist cloth.

● If your child won't cooperate with this, or if you can't remove the particle, cover the eye with a gauze pad taped in place and see a doctor immediately.

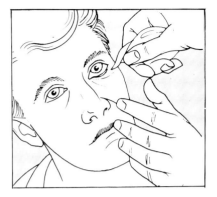

In the case of small foreign bodies in the eye, *put the child under a good light and lift off the particle using the moistened tip of a clean handkerchief or tissue.*

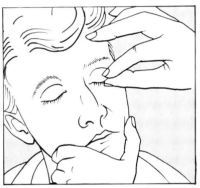

If the particle is stuck *to the undersurface of the upper lid, gently hold the lid and, with the child looking down, rub it gently over the lower lid. If this does not work, place a matchstick in the fold of the upper lid and pull the eyelid over it. You should then be able to remove the particle with the moistened tip of a handkerchief.*

ACID AND CAUSTIC BURNS

If acid or any other caustic substance *has found its way into the eye, hold the child's head under cold running water for several seconds. Make sure the child blinks and opens the eyes while you are doing this. Transfer the child to hospital immediately, continuing to wash the eye if possible during the journey.*

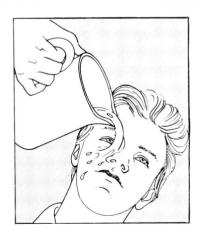

FROSTBITE AND HYPOTHERMIA

FROSTBITE

Frostbite occurs when the skin freezes. It usually affects the nose, cheeks, ears, fingers, and toes. Frostbitten skin turns glossy white or grayish-yellow and feels numb. Sometimes blisters appear. If severe frostbite is not treated, the child goes into shock.

First aid for frostbite involves warming the frozen part—against your body until you reach shelter, and in warm (not hot) water once you come indoors. You can also cover the frozen part with warm towels. Give the child a warm nonalcoholic drink, unless the child is unconscious. Stop the warming treatment as soon as the skin looks flushed. If toes or fingers are affected, separate them with clean cloths, and keep affected limbs raised. Call a doctor immediately. Be sure not to rub frostbitten skin and not to apply heat or hot water to it.

You can help avoid frostbite by making sure that your child's clothing and footwear are dry, warm, and not too tight, and that as much of the body as possible is protected.

HYPOTHERMIA

Hypothermia occurs when the child's body temperature goes down too far, and it too can be fatal. Cold weather, wet clothing, and immersion in water can bring it on quickly. A child with hypothermia shivers, stumbles, looks exhausted or drowsy, and has trouble speaking.

TREATING HYPOTHERMIA

● Bring the child into a warm room immediately, remove all wet or cold clothing, and warm the child with your own body heat, by wrapping the child in blankets, or by placing the child in a tub of warm (not hot) water.

● Give warm, nonalcoholic drinks, unless the child is unconscious.

● Check for frostbite and shock and watch to make sure that the child doesn't stop breathing.

Hypothermia and frostbite (right) *are both serious medical conditions requiring instant and effective medical attention. Prevention is better than cure though and young children should always be very warmly dressed if they are going to be outdoors in windy or cold weather.*

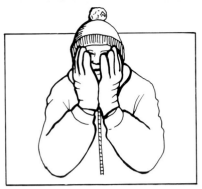

Very young children are vulnerable to frostbite and hypothermia. *Both conditions are serious and require instant and effective medical attention. Frost-bitten parts can be warmed gently, but not rubbed, with gloved hands until medical assistance arrives. Prevention is better than cure though and young children should always be very warmly dressed if they are going to be outdoors in windy or cold weather.*

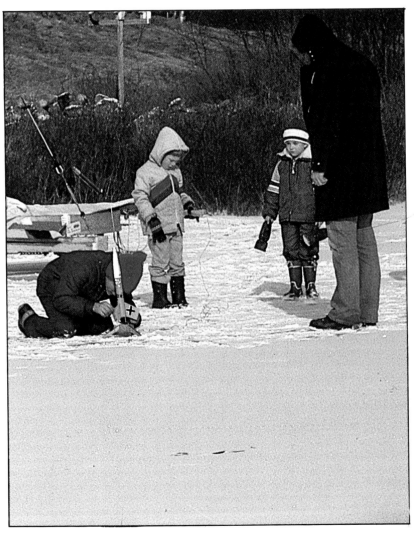

75

INSECT BITES AND STINGS

Many insects and other small creatures bite and sting, but few cause serious problems. The insects described below can cause a health hazard.

BEE, WASP, OR HORNET STING
Few of us escape being stung by a bee or wasp at some point in our lives. Teaching your child to treat these insects with caution and respect will reduce the number of stings he or she receives. The sting injects a venom that causes a few hours of swelling, redness, and sharp pain.

SCORPIONS
Native mainly to the Southwest, scorpions inject venom through a stinger in the tail. The sting site feels intensely painful, and your child develops nausea, vomiting, stomach pain, and may go into shock. Treat as for spider bites. Avoid scorpions on camping trips by shaking out boots and clothes before putting them on in the morning.

Tarantulas and poisonous centipedes bite only very rarely in the United States.

SPIDERS
Two spiders native to the United States, the black widow and the brown recluse, have bites that are dangerous to humans, especially children. Symptoms of black widow bite include severe pain, sweating, nausea, cramps and breathing difficulty. The bite of the brown recluse forms an open ulcer at the bite and causes general pain and nausea.

TREATING SPIDER BITES

● Get medical help immediately.

● Always keep the bitten part below the level of the heart to slow the flow of the poison.

● If the bite is on an arm or leg, put a constricting band on the limb between the bite and the heart. Make the band loose enough to slip a finger underneath. Remove after 30 minutes.

● An ice bag or cold compress eases the pain and swelling at the bite.

TREATING BEE, WASP, AND HORNET STINGS

● Use your fingers or tweezers to remove the stinger if present.

● Apply calamine lotion, antihistamine cream, or a poultice of baking soda and water.

● If the sting is on the mouth, have your child suck an ice cube. Watch for a dangerous swelling of the throat tissues that may cause breathing difficulty.

● If there are multiple stings, or if you note any signs of breathing difficulty or shock, get emergency medical help immediately. Bee stings can cause a fatal form of allergic shock. Have a child with other allergies tested for this problem.

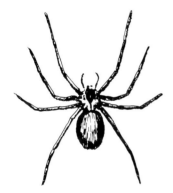

Brown recluse spider

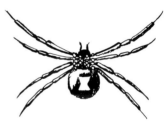

Black widow spider with the hourglass on its underside

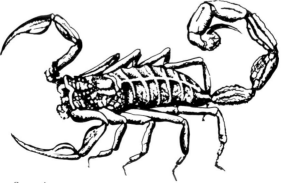

Scorpion

NOSEBLEEDS

Nosebleeds are common among children and are generally not serious. The nose is full of blood vessels and bleeds easily if injured by a fall or blow to the face. Nosebleeds can also be caused by inserting foreign objects into the nose (including fingers) and excessive noseblowing during a cold or allergy attack. Sometimes, however, there is no obvious reason for a nosebleed in an otherwise healthy child.

FOREIGN OBJECTS IN NOSE
If there is an object up the child's nose that cannot be blown out with both nostrils open, see your doctor. Such objects can usually be removed by the doctor with a specially designed instrument. Do not try to remove sharp objects lodged in the nose; get emergency help.

BROKEN NOSE
A broken nose will redden, swell up, bleed heavily, and sometimes appear flattened or pushed to one side. Give first aid as for nosebleeds and get medical help immediately.

FREQUENT OR PROLONGED NOSEBLEEDS
Some children develop swollen blood vessels in the nasal septum that rupture easily, causing frequent nosebleeds. An ear, nose, and throat specialist may be able to shrink the swollen vessels by the application of cauterizing chemicals.

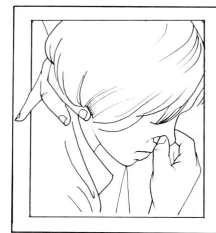

TREATMENT

A child with a nosebleed should be supported with his head forwards (rather than backwards, which may be the instinctive reaction) with the nostrils pinched gently together. If bleeding continues for more than ten minutes or so, an icepack or cold compress should be applied to the nose.

POISON IVY, POISON OAK, AND POISON SUMAC

Poison ivy, poison oak, and poison sumac release irritating oils on contact. An allergic reaction on the skin develops within a few hours, leading to a burning itch, redness, and blisters. Your child may also develop fever and nausea, especially if contact was over a wide area of skin or if the child is liable to suffer from allergies in general.

Prevent exposure to these plants by dressing your child in long sleeves and pants when the child is going out to play in woody areas. Teach your child to identify and avoid these plants.

POISON IVY
Poison ivy grows as a small shrub or a vine. You can recognize it by its glossy leaves, which always grow in threes off a central stem. It grows in woody areas throughout the United States except in some parts of the West Coast.

POISON OAK
Poison oak looks much like poison ivy, but the leaves are broader and have more scalloped edges. It grows mainly in California and adjoining states.

POISON SUMAC
Poison sumac (also called swamp sumac and poison elder) is a woody shrub that grows up to 25 feet tall. Its long, thin leaves are grouped in rows along thin branches. Poison sumac is common in the eastern United States.

TREATING POISON IVY, POISON OAK, AND POISON SUMAC

● Undress your child and wash the skin thoroughly with soap and water. Wash contaminated clothes.

● Apply rubbing alcohol to the exposed area.

● Spread calamine lotion over the rash to soothe the itch.

● See your doctor if the rash does not clear up after a few days or if your child has a more severe reaction.

POISONING AND DRUG OVERDOSE

Many children die each year from poisoning and accidental drug overdose. The typical household contains dozens of poisons, among them detergents, paint, adhesives, gasoline, ammonia, bleach, hair preparations, perfume, drain cleaners, toilet bowl cleaners, insecticides, and medicines. Many backyard plants, such as delphinium, lily-of-the-valley, and most toadstools, are poisonous if eaten. Small children are most likely to be victims of poisoning because they are endlessly inquisitive, instinctively put things into their mouths, and lack the judgment and experience to distinguish poisons and dangerous drugs from other substances. But even older children can mistakenly ingest a poison or drug thinking it is something else.

The best way to combat poisoning is by prevention.

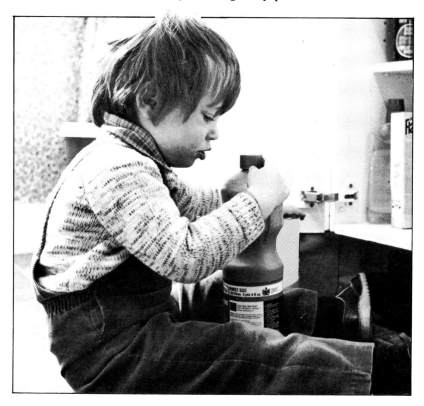

THE FIRST AID CABINET

Keep all your medicines together in one place, preferably in a wall-mounted cabinet positioned high on the wall, out of the reach of young children. Choose a well-designed cabinet that is awkward to open, or, better still, one that can be locked shut. If necessary explain to your child that the medicines are as dangerous to you as they are to them.

POISONING TREATMENT

For Poisoning with Petroleum Products, Bleach, Alkalis, or Acids

● Do not induce vomiting.

● Give your child one or two glasses of milk to drink. If there are burns around the mouth, also give five teaspoons of activated charcoal (available at drugstores) mixed in a glass of water.

● Treat for shock. Get emergency medical care.

For Other Poisons

● Give milk or water to dilute the poison.

● Try to induce vomiting by giving one tablespoon of syrup of ipecac or sticking one or two fingers down the child's throat.

● If the child is unconscious, do not induce vomiting. Keep the child's head down to stop vomit from being inhaled. Treat for shock. Get emergency medical care.

FIRST AID FOR POISONING AND DRUG OVERDOSE

If you suspect that your child has ingested a poison or drug, look for an empty poison container, sudden pain or illness, stains or burns around the lips and mouth, and chemical odor on clothes or breath. Other symptoms can include vomiting, dizziness, convulsions, sleepiness, and coma. Contact your poison control center immediately, and get emergency medical help. Save the empty container or a sample of vomit for analysis.

Store all dangerous chemicals and cleaning fluids (left) where children cannot reach them.

SHOCK

Shock is a state of bodily depression that follows an injury or severe illness. Untreated, it can be fatal, even if the injury that caused it would not have been. Shock can be caused by serious wounds and blood loss; by loss of body fluids through vomiting and diarrhea; by burns; by poisoning and drug overdose; by heatstroke; and, especially in children, by emotional trauma. Shock can also be part of a severe allergic reaction.

Shock must be identified quickly and handled carefully. Early symptoms include pale, bluish, or mottled skin; nausea; weakness; and rapid pulse and breathing. In later stages of shock the pupils may be dilated and the child loses consciousness and feels cold to the touch. *It is extremely important in cases of shock to get medical help immediately.* To be safe, always treat a seriously injured child for shock.

TREATING SHOCK

The first goal in giving first aid for shock is to treat the immediate cause. Stop any bleeding, bandage wounds, and give CPR if necessary. Comfort your child and have the child lie down in a comfortable position—on the side or back is best. Do not move the child, however, if you think there may be a neck or back injury. Prop up the feet above the head; this helps the child's circulation. An unconscious child should be placed on his or her side to keep the airway open.

It is a good idea to cover the child with a blanket or coat, but don't put too many layers on—overheating can be dangerous in shock. Do not give any fluids. *Summon help immediately.*

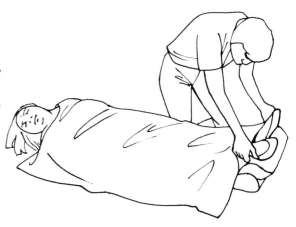

A child suffering from shock will have some or all of the following symptoms: clammy skin and sweating, pale complexion, shallow pulse, irregular breathing and enlarged pupils. The casualty should be placed on his back with the legs raised. Tight clothes should be loosened and the child kept warm.

SPLINTERS AND BLISTERS

SPLINTERS

Removing splinters is one of the important parental arts. Follow the steps listed here.

REMOVING SPLINTERS

● Large splinters can usually be pulled right out with your fingers or tweezers. Wash the spot with rubbing alcohol.

● Splinters trapped under the skin may be hard to see. Direct a good light on the spot. Stain the area with iodine or food coloring; the splinter will absorb the dye and show up better.

● Have your child numb the area with ice.

● Sterilize a sewing needle and tweezers in a flame or by dipping them in rubbing alcohol.

● Gently prick open the skin with the needle. Squeeze behind the splinter to push it forward. Grasp the end with the tweezers and remove.

● Wash the area with rubbing alcohol and put a bandage on the spot if asked.

BLISTERS

Blisters are swollen pockets of fluid caused by heat or excessive friction on the skin of the hands and feet. They can be prevented by: Having your child wear gloves to do outside work, such as raking leaves; choosing shoes that fit well and breaking in new shoes gradually; changing socks regularly on long walks or hikes to keep the feet dry.

Blisters need to be kept clean and covered. They can become infected if left untreated.

TREATING BLISTERS

● Do not break the blister if it has not already broken.

● Cover with a clean dressing.

● Put on some padding (a gauze pad or two will do) and tape in place.

SPRAINS, STRAINS & DISLOCATIONS

SPRAINS

When a joint is forcibly stretched beyond its limits there may be tearing and damage around it—a sprain. Children are likely to suffer muscle strains in normal play, but older children who play sports are even more prone to sprained elbows, turned ankles, and wrenched knees.

TREATING SPRAINS

● Keep your child off the injured limb. Elevate the limb to reduce swelling.

● Wrap the joint in an elasticized bandage. Bind firmly, but not so tight as to cut off circulation.

● A cold compress or an ice bag further reduces swelling.

● See your doctor or a sports-injury specialist for excessive swelling or a very painful sprain.

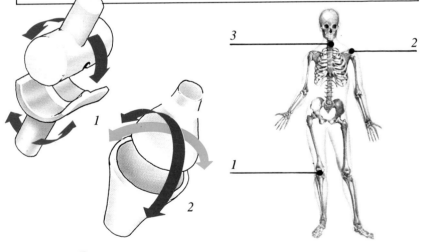

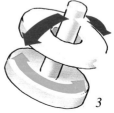

Synovial joints are particularly vulnerable to sprains and strains. The three main types are: (1) Hinge joints, found at the knee, elbow and fingers. (2) Ball and socket joints, found at the shoulder and hip. (3) Pivot joint, found between the first and second vertebrae in the neck.

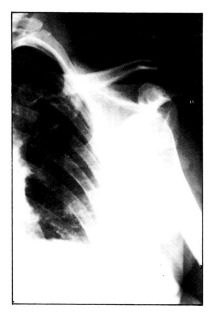

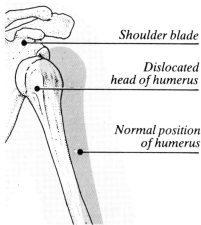

Shoulder blade

Dislocated
head of humerus

Normal position
of humerus

The flexibility of the shoulder joint *means that it may become dislocated with relatively little force.*

STRAINS

Strains are stretched or pulled muscles. These can usually be treated at home with warm, wet compresses and rest of the injured muscle.

DISLOCATIONS

Dislocations occur when a joint is separated or pushed out of its normal position. Shoulder and finger dislocations are the most common, but the jaw, elbow, hip, and knee can also be wrenched out of alignment. The injured joint usually looks deformed and there is swelling and a bruise later on. Medical help is always needed to treat a dislocation.

TREATING DISLOCATIONS

● Get medical help. It is often difficult to distinguish between a dislocation and a fracture, so if you are in doubt as to what kind of injury your child has and have to move the child yourself, treat it as a fracture.

● Don't try to realign the joint yourself. This is best done by your doctor or a specialist.

● Keep your child quiet and off the injured joint until you get help.

SUNBURN AND SUNSTROKE

SUNBURN
Sunburn occurs when radiation from the sun (or from a sunlamp or tanning lamp) makes the skin turn painfully red and sore. Children burn very easily, especially those with fair skin. The best way to prevent sunburn is to keep your child's exposure to direct sunlight at a minimum. (Even half an hour in full sun may be too much for some children.) Make sure the child wears a brimmed hat and is well-covered by clothes. Wherever the skin is exposed, apply a sunscreen lotion that contains PABA, and put more lotion on when the child comes back from swimming. Be extra careful on the beach or in a boat, since the cool breeze may fool you into thinking that protection is not needed. Sunburn takes six to twelve hours to develop, and skin that feels cool to the touch in the afternoon can turn bright red in the evening.

Once burning has occurred, keep the child completely out of the sun until the skin heals. You can cool the skin with warm (not cold) water and let it dry in the air. Calamine lotion and aspirin or acetaminophen may give some relief. The skin hurts if anything touches it, so let the child wear smooth, light clothes. Give your child plenty to drink to allow the skin to build up moisture lost through burning.

In a case of severe sunburn, blisters form on the skin. They may become infected if they burst. The child should be examined by a doctor.

SUNSTROKE
Heat from the sun, a fire, or any other source can produce danger-ous physical reactions. When the weather is hot and humid, you can help your child avoid heat reactions by giving him or her plenty to drink, by not allowing too much exercise in the sun, by dressing the child in loose clothes, and by running a fan or air conditioner in the house.

HEAT EXHAUSTION
Heat exhaustion makes your child feel weak and dizzy, with clammy, sweaty skin, and sometimes with muscle cramps. Have the child lie down, unclothed, in a cool, shaded room, with the feet raised. Run a fan or air conditioner and put cool, moist cloths over the child's body. For the next hour, give the child frequent sips from a glass containing water mixed with one teaspoon of salt.

However, if the child vomits, he or she must be taken to a hospital where salt water can be given intravenously.

HEAT STROKE

Heat stroke is a derangement of the body's temperature controls, and it can be fatal. *Sunstroke* is a common form of heat stroke that includes sunburn symptoms. The sunburn may be severe, with blistering. The warning signs of sunstroke are exhaustion, irritability, headache, dizziness, and muscle cramps. Full sunstroke occurs when the body temperature rises to 104°F (40°C) or more. The child is restless, confused, or even semiconscious, with a rapid pulse and dry, flushed skin.

TREATING SUNSTROKE

● Lower the child's temperature without delay. Quickly remove the child's clothes. Wrap the child in a cold, wet sheet, with a fan or air conditioner running, or sponge off the child in a tub half-full of cool water.

● When the child's temperature is down, dry him or her off and call a doctor. You may need to repeat the treatment.

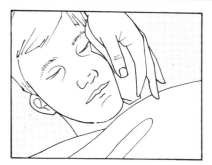

A child suffering from heatstroke should be wrapped in a cold, wet sheet to bring the body temperature down. Create a current of air around the casualty by fanning with a newspaper or other suitable object. Take the child's temperature at regular intervals, and once it has fallen replace the wet sheet with a dry one. If the child is unconscious place him or her in the recovery position and send for medical help.

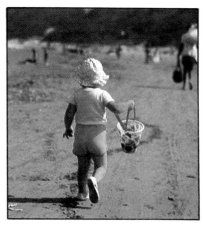

Young children are particularly susceptible to sunburn on the beach or after swimming. Protective clothing and the regular application of a suitable sunscreen lotion to exposed skin should be adequate preventive measures.

YOUR CHILD IN THE HOSPITAL

A hospital stay can be a worrying time for a child. It is hard for any child to leave home and friends and go to an unfamiliar place full of strangers. It is even harder for a sick or injured child, who has the added stress of painful or unpleasant symptoms or medical procedures.

If hospital admission is planned in advance, the parents can talk it over with the child and let the child know what to expect. Most hospitals welcome a visit before the admission so that the child can become familiar with the children's ward and meet some of the staff.

Whether a hospitalization is planned in advance or is sudden and unplanned, a parent's presence can do much to ease the child's anxiety and distress. Most children's units have some accommodation for parents, or can provide a cot next to your child's bed. Often the hospital food service will provide meals for parents at additional cost.

If parents are unable to stay with their children, it helps for them to visit as much as possible. They should tell the child when they are leaving and when they are coming back, so the child can take comfort in looking forward to their return. Many hospitals will allow the parents to appoint a relative or friend to stay with the child if they themselves cannot stay.

Children come to hospitals for investigation and treatment of illness, but they continue to have all the other needs of children as well—for feeding, washing, toileting, playing, amusement, friendship, and love. Parents can take care of these needs just as they do at home, sometimes with the help of the nurses. All members of the hospital staff—doctors, nurses, technicians, play therapists, and support staff—have important roles to play in helping your child get well. But your hospitalized child still needs *you,* more than ever. You and your family can work with the hospital staff so that your child gets plenty of parental love and attention during medical treatment.

It takes a while for children to return to their usual behavior when they come home from hospital. Young children often become clinging and refuse to let their parents out of sight. Children of any age may be quiet and withdrawn, or quick to cry. Often the normal sleeping pattern is disturbed, and reversion to previous habits like thumb-sucking and bed-wetting may occur. Parents can help the child feel confident and secure again by being patient and understanding.

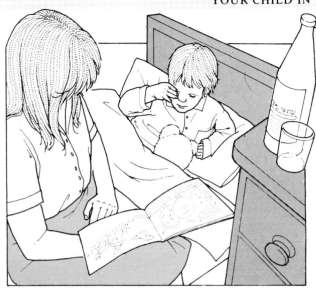

You will want to visit your child in hospital regularly (left). Establish what the visiting hours are and always reassure your child that you will come back as often and for as long as possible and that the hospital stay won't last for ever.

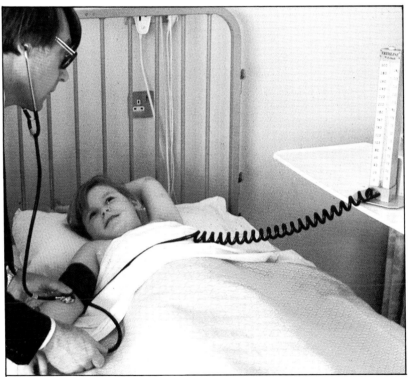

Measuring blood pressure may be one of the routine tests that a child is given during a stay in hospital.

Many hospitals have special children's wards and facilities for parents to stay overnight.

A GUIDE TO MEDICAL TERMS

Many medical words are derived from Latin and Greek. If you know the meaning of the Latin and Greek parts of the words, it is easy to interpret many medical words that at first sight seem complex. A selection is listed below. The position of the hyphen shows whether the word part is placed at the beginning or the end of the word.

A

a-, an-: a lack of, an absence of
ab-: away from
ad-: toward, near to
-emia: of the blood
andr-: of the male sex
anti-: against, opposing
-arch-, -arche-: first
arthr-: of a joint
audio-: of hearing, or sound
aut-, auto-: self

B

bi-: two
brady-: slowness

C

-cele: a swelling
-centesis: perforation
chron-: time
-cide: destroyer
contra-: against, opposite
cryo-: cold
-cyte: a cell

D

de-: removal, or loss
derm-: of the skin
dipl-: double
dys:- difficulty, abnormality

E

ec-, ect-: outside, external
-ectomy: surgical removal
em-, en-: inside, internal
end-: inner, within
enter-: of the intestine
epi-: upon, over
erythr:- red
ex-, exo-: outside of, outer
extra-: outside, beyond

F

fibr-: of fibrous tissue

G

-genic: producing
-gram: record, trace
-graph: a device that records

H

hem-: of the blood
hepat-: of the liver
hetero-: dissimilar
homeo-: alike
hydr-: of water, or fluid
hyp-, hypo-: deficiency in, lack of
hyper-: excess of

I

-iasis: a disease state
inter-: between
intra-: inside
-itis: inflammation

L

laparo-: of the abdomen or loins
leuc-, leuk-: white
-lysis: breaking up

M

macro-: large
mal-: disorder, abnormality
-mania: compulsion, obsession
mast-: of the breast
megal-: abnormally large
-megaly: abnormal enlargement
mes-: middle
met-, meta-: (a) change, e.g., metabolism; (b) distant, e.g., metastasis
micro-: small
myo-, my-: of the muscles
myelo-: of the spine

N

nephr:- of the kidneys
neur-: of the nerves

O

-oma: a tumor
-osis: a disease state
ost-: of bone
-otomy: a surgical examination

P

pan-: all
para-: (a) near, e.g., paramedian; (b) like, e.g. paratyphoid; (c) abnormal, e.g., paresthesia
path-: of disease
-pathy: disease
-penia: deficiency
peri-: near, around
-philia: craving, love for
phleb-: of the veins
-plasia: formation
-phlegia: paralysis
pneu-: of respiration
-poiesis: formation
poly-: many

pre-: (a) before, e.g., prenatal; (b) in front of, e.g., prevertebral
pro-: before, in front of
proct-: of the anus and rectum

R

rhin-: of the nose

S

-stasis: standing still
sub-: below

T

tox-: poisonous
trans-: through, across
-trophy: growth, development

V

vas-: a vessel

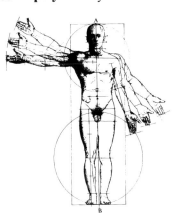

THE FIRST AID KIT

Dealing with childhood illnesses and injuries is made easier and safer if you keep emergency medical supplies handy in a first aid kit. One large kit should be kept at home, and another in your car,

FIRST AID KIT FOR A FAMILY OF FOUR

1 cotton balls
2 elastic bandage
  and butterfly closures
3 stretch gauze bandage
4 gauze swabs
5 antacid
6 Epsom salts
7 calamine lotion
8 aspirin
9 children's aspirin
10 acetaminophen
11 salt tablets
12 adhesive tape
13 assorted adhesive bandages
14 sterile pads for bandaging
15 sharp blunt-ended scissors
16 lipscreen
17 cotton swabs
18 petroleum jelly
19 analgesic tablets
20 antacid tablets
21 antibiotic ointment
22 set measuring spoons
23 tweezers
24 family thermometers

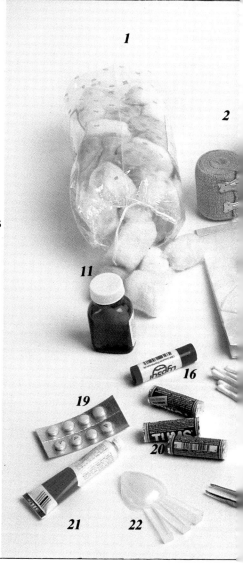

van, boat, or trailer. Make sure that you keep the kit fully stocked and that family members and babysitters know where it is kept.

Various types and sizes of complete kits can be purchased at medical supply houses and large pharmacies, but you can also create your own kit. Fill a watertight box with the items listed here.

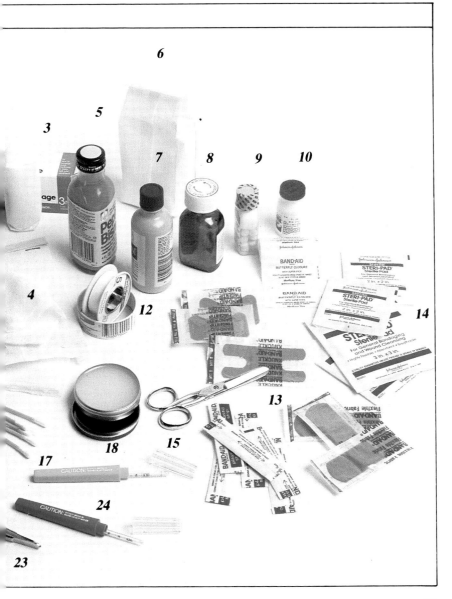

INDEX

EMERGENCY NUMBERS

Post a copy of this list of emergency phone numbers near every phone in your house.

Police	
Fire Department	
Rescue Squad or Ambulance	
Hospital Emergency	
Poison Control Center	
Health Department	
Pediatrician	Home
Family Doctor	Home
Alternate Doctor	Home
Dentist	Home
All-Night Drugstore	
Father's Work Number	
Mother's Work Number	
Neighbors	
Taxi